Children are...
Images of Grace

A Pediatrician's Trilogy of Faith, Hope, and Love

DIANE M. KOMP, M.D.

ZondervanPublishingHouse
Grand Rapids, Michigan

A Division of HarperCollins*Publishers*

Requests for information should be addressed to:

ZondervanPublishingHouse
Grand Rapids, Michigan 49530

ISBN: 0-310-20699-5

Interior design by Sue Vandenberg Koppenol

Printed in the United States of America

96 97 98 99 00 01 02 /❖DH/ 10 9 8 7 6 5 4 3 2 1

To my patients:
"I love these little people;
and it is not a slight thing when they,
who are so fresh from God, love us."

—Charles Dickens, *The Old Curiosity Shop*

Contents

Preface

Several years ago one of my former professors posed a challenge to me. "What do you collect?" he asked. He, a world traveler, filled his home with priceless relics of his many visits to the Far East. I don't collect objects of art as he does. I collect stories. Stories about children are my treasure.

My intention was to wait until I retired from medical practice as a pediatric cancer specialist before I committed these treasures to the printed page. For many years I entered stories into my computer's memory or scribbled them onto paper placemats at assorted restaurants. Organizing them seemed like a suitable project to keep me out of mischief when it comes time for younger clinicians to carry the beeper.

Over the years I have used a number of these stories to illustrate sermons, enliven adult Sunday school programs, or even punctuate private conversation. But there came an urgency that made me change my time frame. One Sunday I told the story of my own spiritual journey to a church group. My listeners had assumed that I had always been a Christian. It was their pastor who said, "You've got to start writing about this. The way you tell the story, you could even convince unbelieving clergy." Somehow I had been naïve enough to think that unbelieving scientists were the toughest to persuade about spiritual truth.

Ken Norris's words forced me to consider publication earlier than I had planned, and led me to *Theology Today*. Editor Hugh Kerr's prompt response to my query included a copy of the memorial service program for the grandson of his best friend, a boy who died from leukemia. The boy had experienced visions similar to those of the children described in my essay. Many essays later, it was "Tim" Kerr who said, "Di, it's time for the book." "The book" turned into a trilogy, yet each of the three is quite difference in style and content.

When the trilogy was complete, a psychiatrist-friend asked me to summarize each of my books in one sentence each. That seemed easy: *A Window to Heaven* is about children and death. *A Child Shall Lead Them* is about children and life. And *Rebekah's Twins* is about mothers. "Wrong!" my friend replied. "*Window* is about you and the children. *Child* is about you and the children. And *Rebekah's Twins* is about you and the children. You need to understand that." I'll leave it to you, the reader, to decide what these stories say about you as well.

In telling these stories, I found it wise to change names and minor details. Whenever possible and appropriate, I consulted the children's parents for the stories in *Window* and *Child*. The story form of *Rebekah's Twins* required a different and more rigorous approach to protect the privacy of adults. We adults would like to be "reliable witnesses" like the children but we are often reluctant to reveal our own stories since we do not share the children's lack of regret.

Thus, none of the seven stories in *Rebekah's Twins* is a "straight line" that follows one family's journey. The characters are composites, blended from thousands of families I've had the privilege to know during a career that spans more than thirty years. Here, I not only changed names, places and details wherever necessary, but also added imagined elements and historical events to enhance readability.

In *Rebekah's Twins*, I invited "hostesses" for the mothers I know to show you how profoundly true these stories really are. In fact, it was these biblical hostesses—Rebekah and Rahab, Hannah and Hagar, Mary and Martha, Tamar and Moses's mother—who suggested which stories from my practice I should share. I changed the name of Moses's mother from Jochebed to "Elena" to better suit the ethnic context of my story and avoid confusion with Jonadab, a villain in Tamar's biblical story. Some of the biblical models suggested a particular ethnic locus or social construct from my own world to frame the story. I intend no racial or cultural stereotype by the choices I made.

Before you draw conclusions about sickness, death, the meaning of life—even the meaning of suffering—let these various images come out of the shadows and into your full view. Let all of these families, ancient and modern, speak for themselves. Even let them disturb you. Let them point to your broken places if you want to learn of hope and grace. Glimpse their special portion of human experience and open your ears so you can hear some of God's finest whispers. Most of these families are just like yours and mine: in need of grace for strength to be made perfect in weakness.

It is my hope that these stories will encourage you to be a bearer of grace to all families, sharing in their suffering. And what you hear from me through these several witnesses, entrust to faithful people, especially those who will be able to teach others as well.

Diane M. Komp
New Haven, CT
May, 1995

A Window to Heaven

Prologue:

Journey to Disbelief

With three or more people there is something bold in the air: direct things get said which would frighten two people alone. . . . To be three is to be in public, you feel safe.
ELIZABETH BOWEN, THE HOUSE IN PARIS

A few years ago I shared a compartment on a railroad train to Frankfurt with an elderly German widow and a Greek auto mechanic. Busy knitting needles punctuated the widow's story as she anticipated a visit to her beloved grandchildren. The Greek gentleman was revisiting the village where he had learned his professional trade years earlier. Both of my fellow passengers were curious about a German-speaking American.

I told them that I had traveled to Marburg to meet with a group of medical students who wanted to discuss the relevance of faith to the practice of medicine. They stared at me in disbelief. Surely they had misunderstood me. Perhaps my German wasn't as fluent as it initially sounded. To them I looked and acted nothing like their image of a professor of medicine. They were certain, however, that I was American. What other genre of middle-aged female would board a train in Germany dressed in blue jeans and Nike sneakers? Perhaps I wasn't talking about *German* medical students. One hears all sorts of things about the religiosity of Americans.

But they had heard me correctly.

The animated Greek groped for words in a language he hadn't used for thirty years: "The only verse in the Bible that our Greek doctors know is the one about the thirty pieces of silver. But they've raised the price. They'd hardly settle for that low of a fee anymore. Why, the chiropractor in our village only charges you the most you can afford to pay!" I resisted the temptation to ask him how he set his fees in his auto service station.

The widow's concerns were more profound: "Our doctors in Germany don't believe in God" was her sad opinion. "When my husband was dying of cancer, I asked our family practitioner if he believed in God. He said no. I asked him how he could help someone to die if he did not believe himself. He just looked away."

This German family doctor reminded me of Albert Camus' fictional French physician, Dr. Rieux. In *The Plague*, Rieux worked tirelessly and compassionately, fighting against an absurd situation (bubonic plague). He saw no higher explanation, only a biological reality. In attending to a friend on his deathbed, the doctor

> . . . could only stand, unavailing, on the shore, empty-handed and sick at heart, unarmed and helpless yet again under the onset of calamity. And thus, when the end came, the tears that blinded Rieux's eyes were tears of impotence; and he did not see Tarrou roll over, face to the wall, and die. . . . The doctor could not tell if Tarrou had found peace, now that it was over, but for himself he had a feeling that no peace was possible to him henceforth, any more than there can be an

14

armistice for a mother bereaved of her son or for a
man who buries his friend.[1]

The German and Greek practitioners that my fellow
passengers encountered are typical of the average Western
physician. Although I know physicians of deep personal faith
both in Europe and in America, they are a minority in my
profession.

Like the fictional Rieux, most doctors working in a
medically privileged society feel unfruitful when our efforts fail
and we cannot cure the disease. These feelings of powerless-
ness negatively affect not only how doctors interpret our discipline of medicine but also how we approach the bedside of
human beings we attend.

For many young doctors who begin their careers from
a perspective of faith in God, the path of medical education
becomes a journey to disbelief. When I started my career in
pediatrics, I vacillated between being an agnostic and an atheist—though I spent little time considering exactly where my
beliefs fit. Like many of my fellow students, I sought the help
of my professors for career guidance, and they were most willing to offer what advice they could from their own experience.

When I faced my first patient who would die (a young
woman my own age with end-stage kidney disease), I asked my
clinical mentor how we as young doctors could deal with our
feelings about so-called "innocent suffering." He responded
that the answer was *not* to attempt to deal with feelings but
simply to do our work and concentrate on that.

Hard work is a good tonic for untamed and uneasy
feelings. His advice seemed good because it appeared to help
me through the ordeal. I learned from him to keep my feelings
about patients as numb as possible. One of the side effects of

15

this approach was that my faith began to slip away with each passing child.

Over the years I have come to the conclusion that dramatic conversion to disbelief is rare. More often, faith dies from disuse, atrophy, a failure to be exercised. Such was my experience. I settled for an ersatz-existentialist's resolution and decided not to attempt to find a meaning in suffering. I only sought to fight against it.

A recent study reveals that few American medical students find anything in their educational process to support and sustain the idealism with which they began their studies. Something about the educational process robs them of their original passion for service and substitutes a different, more self-oriented motivation. A young person who previously identified with the sufferer moves to a position where there is a seemingly unbridgeable distance between patient and physician.

The chaplain of a medical school interviewed clinical faculty members to determine how these experienced physicians coped with the extraordinary stresses of their work. He quotes an internist who is representative of his colleagues. This doctor described how he has learned to cope with the absurdity of serious illness: "I no longer assume the responsibility for the successful outcome or failure, if the success or failure is determined by the impotency of medicine as opposed to my mistake. I do not establish friendships with my patients; there is no socializing. I learned that very early on."[2]

Thus, my own story is not the only one of a physician whose early idealistic and religious convictions were to be derailed during medical education. My journey begins in derailment but does not end there.

1

A Choir of Angels

My strategy of remaining emotionally detached from my patients simply did not work. Taking care of children is quite different from treating adults. Internists and surgeons may get away with keeping their distance, but for a pediatrician treating children with chronic diseases it is not a viable option. Whether atheists, agnostics, or firm believers, pediatricians must learn to listen to our young patients if we would gain their cooperation and practice something more communicative than veterinary medicine.

One of the bittersweet privileges of caring for children with cancer is that you grow to love them and bask in that love returned. We rarely see this form of love returned on this earth. It is unconditional. Part of that love entails, on occasion, the sharing of the road toward death.

As a young "post-Christian" doctor, I did not pretend to have any handy theological solutions to people's existential dilemmas, but I could be a friend on the way. Many times I listened politely to parents who groped for God in their most painful hour. I respected them all for their journeys, but I heard no convincing evidence in their revelations that challenged my way of thinking. I always assumed that if I were to believe, it would take the testimony of reliable witnesses. I mistrusted anyone who might have culturally determined expectations about death or an I-can't-afford-not-to-believe view of the hereafter.

In the early years of the 1970s, brave parents helped me implement a home death program in a rural area of the South. As a cancer specialist for children at the time, I visited my patients at home. Sometimes they had physical pain but rarely did they seem afraid. In their homes, I was the guest and they were clearly the hosts. Children accurately reported their medical condition in this environment, since they felt in control. With encouragement and support, many families found they could manage pain and other dreaded complications of terminal cancer. If the children did need hospitalization for comfort, they themselves felt free to suggest it. If they preferred to die at home, we made it possible long before hospice services were more generally available.

In their homes, children would ceremoniously wipe the dust from my black doctor's bag and swear that they would not report me to the AMA for making house calls. My young patients and I would discuss what type of examination was appropriate, what tests might be useful, and they themselves determined the limits. I rarely used the syringes, needles, and blood test tubes in my bag. Tea in the kitchen with the rest of the family followed the visit to the patient's room, for the brothers and sisters—those who would live on—needed special attention as well.

Most children who die in this situation do not pass from this life without prior warning. Often parents of children at home or nursing staff of hospitalized patients could alert me in time to be at the bedside for that moment. The first time I sat by a child dying of cancer, I sat at her bed from a sense of duty rather than in anticipation of joy.

Today many children with leukemia are cured, but this was not the case when Anna first became sick. There were periods of time that she was disease-free over the five years she received treatment, but she faced the end of her life at the age of seven. Before she died, Anna mustered the final energy to sit up in her hospital bed and say: "The angels—they're so beautiful! Mommy, can you see them? Do you hear their singing? I've never heard such beautiful singing!" Then she lay back on her pillow and died.

Her parents reacted as if they had received the most precious gift in the world. The hospital chaplain in attendance was more comfortable with the psychological than with the spiritual. He beat a hasty retreat to leave the existentialist doctor alone with the grieving family. Together we contemplated a spiritual mystery that transcended our combined understanding and experience. For weeks to follow, this thought stuck in my head: *Have I found a reliable witness?*

Everytime I hear the angel prologue to Boito's opera *Mephistopheles*, I think of Anna and the other "angels" who brought their oncologist back to the life of faith. My encounter with these children changed my life. Other stalled journeys of faith have been resumed. I write these stories as a witness to these children and their parents, just as they have been faithful witnesses to me.

Several years ago, I had the opportunity to tell the story of Anna's vision of angels at a church conference. One participant was particularly overcome by the story and ran out of the room in tears. His reaction seemed to be a very personal one rather than generalized sadness about death in children. Later in the day, he returned and explained to the group why he had been so profoundly affected by Anna's story.

Twenty years before, Walter had personally witnessed a tragic accident. A driver parked a beer truck on an incline adjacent to a local pub while he made his delivery. The brakes of the truck were somehow faulty. Just as Walter walked out the barroom door and reached the street, the truck began to move unattended. It accelerated down a steep hill toward a mother and young child.

Walter anticipated what would happen to the child if the truck did not stop. He tried to catch it in time to put on the emergency brake but his efforts failed, in part, because the large amount of alcohol in his system impeded his reflexes. In fact, he was at that time an established alcoholic.

His worst fears were realized, and the child was fatally pinned against the wall. In his alcoholic stupor, he thought he saw the child's head surrounded by light and heard her last words to her mother: "Don't worry, Mommy. I'll be okay."

The shock and guilt he felt precipitated a two-week drinking binge, but his sense of a supernatural presence at the moment of her death led him to seek effective help for his alcoholism.

Can there be anything good about the death of a child? As Walter told his story, I remembered a comment that he had made earlier in the group's discussion—a comment that had led me to tell Anna's story to begin with. Walter said something to the effect that children are important in God's redemptive plan for us.

Walter's reflection is consistent with the words of Jesus, who often pointed to children when he required an apt metaphor for the kingdom of heaven. Jesus rarely used adults as role models for spiritual maturity.

Like Walter I must ask myself what my life would be like today if I were not privileged to know these dying children. Would I have found that window to heaven that later defined the most important experiences of my life?

2

Hearts Unsure,
Hearts Untroubled

*To have his path made clear for him is the aspiration of
every human being in our beclouded and tempestuous
existence.*

JOSEPH CONRAD, *THE MIRROR OF THE SEA*

I cannot report that the choir of angels resulted in a
dramatic conversion experience for me or in an instant
resumption of the traditional beliefs I had abandoned. For me
it was a prologue. That experience posed important questions
that hinted at the answers that might follow.

A prologue tunes our ears to the composer's desired
cadences and relegates former dominating themes to less
active memory. My heart remained unsure when I left Anna's
hospital room, but my ear had definitely been retuned.

Although physicians do not generally recognize it, our
ears are continuously being retuned. We take pride that our
observations are objective and complete. We believe that we
hear and tell the whole story. The fact is that since it is a

human listener who is recording the facts, the "truth" is fil-
tered through personal experience. If a "fact" does not make
sense to us, we may not even hear it.

Once I caught this cadence of old familiar truth I realized that, in my acquired "deafness," I might not know everything about my patients that was important to learn. With the
retuning of my ear I became a more objective, less censoring
listener.

My introduction to Mary Beth came somewhat later.
She was six years old when I diagnosed her cancer. After a
brief period out of the hospital, her disease recurred. In defer-
ence to her parents' wishes, we did not discuss her worsening
condition in her presence. The change in treatment meant
that I must admit Mary Beth to the hospital shortly before
Christmas. She wasn't afraid of the hospital because she had
made friends with the nurses at the time of her first admission.
The staff planned a holiday party for the children, and Mary
Beth's favorite nurse bought her a red velvet dress to wear.
Mysteriously, the child refused to wear it for reasons she firmly
declined to discuss. Mary Beth was fond of pretty dresses, so
her behavior was very much out of character.

After she completed her treatment, her blood counts
indicated that she was not responding. We discussed the
child's poor prognosis with her family, and discharged Mary
Beth to come back to visit as an outpatient. At the time of a
return visit, her mother confessed that she was baffled by a
dream that the child had shared with her. She asked me what
I thought it meant.

Mary Beth had told her mother of a dream in which
Jesus came to visit her with a grandfather who had died before
the child was born. Together, Jesus and her grandfather told
her of her impending death and encouraged her not to be

afraid. She awoke with the peace and reassurance that she would soon be with Jesus and her grandfather.

She had never met that grandfather but recognized him from family photographs. It was her absolute peace that baffled her mother. Mary Beth died at home on Christmas Eve. She was dressed in her new red velvet dress at the funeral that celebrated her brief life.

Although the dream baffled her mother, it reminded me of my previous experience with Anna and other children. These encounters had opened a window for me that had long been tightly shuttered. I recognized a pattern in their stories that helped me reexamine systems of belief that lay on the other side of the window.

The stories in this book are not based on the type of systematic research that makes scientists feel comfortable and secure. At the same time, being comfy and certain does not necessarily mean that we know all the truth.

Scientists tend to define what we are trying to understand in terms that we already know. This increases our comfort level. We are cautious by temperament. We are reluctant to speak out on any subject until we are certain of it. We hesitate to speak about non-science in a manner that might be misinterpreted as an *ex cathedra* scientific report. We do not know what to do with observations that fall outside our own carefully controlled experiments. When we cannot speak the language of science, we would rather remain silent.

For many years, I did not share these stories of the children in public, but I did allow them to nurture me privately. *Los Angeles Times* journalist Dianne Klein captured this reluctance when she quoted one of my colleagues who has shared similar experiences: "Talking about this with me makes [Dr.] Geni Bennetts a little uncomfortable. She doesn't want to sound like a kook, which she is most certainly not. 'I cannot accept it as science. I accept it as part of life. I have never tried to prove it—or disprove it. I just accept it.'"[1]

The children's experiences did not correspond to anything I learned in medical school, but they did remind me of words I learned in my youth. Jesus intended to dispel the fear and sadness he saw on his disciples' faces:

> Let not your heart be troubled: ye believe in God, believe also in me. In my Father's house are many mansions: if it were not so, I would have told you. I go to prepare a place for you. And if I go and prepare a place for you, I will come again, and receive you unto myself; that where I am, there ye may be also. (John 14:1–3 KJV)

Jesus spoke of an alternative to the unsure, uncertain heart—the heart untroubled. We do not achieve the untroubled heart that he describes by gaining access to more information about the subject we fear. Neither is this peace the result of an intellectual desensitization to painful words and concepts. Theologian Paul Minear interprets this peace simply as a gift:

> The peace is not a vague state of bliss in general, but *his* peace, something belonging to him that he alone can give as a farewell bequest. Nor is it spread on the winds for universal appreciation; it is given only to *his own*, those who belong to him and who are being commissioned to carry on his work. It forever links their work to his, their story to his.[2]

The stories in this book link an ancient story with the children's stories. Rather than medical case reports based on the certainty of what scientists currently understand, they are simply an attempt to be faithful to what I have heard. In this sense, the stories continue Jesus' commissioned work of revealing that there is a realm that we cannot yet fully understand. The greatest gift in my life has been in linking the ancient story and the children's stories to my own. As I accepted the linkage, God was able to minister to my unsure heart with the gift of these hearts untroubled.

3

Something Better Than Near Death

To die is different from what any one supposed.
WALT WHITMAN, LEAVES OF GRASS

Some have linked my work with the so-called "near-death experience." Although the reported near-death experiences bear some superficial similarities to some aspects of these stories of children who would soon die, the differences are more striking.

Most adults who have near-death experiences tell their stories with fear that they will not be believed. The young children who experience these visions, however, are confident that they will be believed. Unlike the adults whom they tell, the children share their stories without a trace of reticence.

If I could use one word to summarize the adult experiences it would be *Aha!* A more apropos summary word for the children would be *Amen.*

For adults, the experience is often spiritually *revolutionary*, a type of conversion experience that puts them on a new road. For children, however, the experience is more spiritually *evolutionary*, progress on an already familiar pathway.

Many adults report vague spiritual beings, but the children are often more specific, naming Jesus or describing angels. Dr. Geni Bennetts tells this story:

> Another boy, a 4-year-old Asian whose family did not practice a Christian faith, had a vision of an angel visiting him and then summoned members of the hospital staff into his room. He thanked each of them for helping him and then said good-bye. Then he lay down and died. . . . He was not upset, not at all. But you can imagine. There wasn't a dry eye on the floor.[1]

Young children with advanced cancer, like adults, report peaceful feelings or seeing light. I have never heard a young child suffering from cancer report seeing a tunnel or darkness. Neither have I heard a child report feeling "out-of-body," nor review their life events. These are common components of near-death experiences.

Many of the reports of near-death experience take place in the setting of clinical death, coma, or another form of brain impairment. The children I am describing report experiences in dreams, visions, or prayer and are infrequently brain dysfunctional at the time.

Developmental psychologists would have us believe that children are less complete than adults and need experience to inform them about the way the world really is. Yet Jesus tells us that we should be like them, these little ones "fresh from God," if we would even begin to understand his Father's love.

Henri Nouwen offers his understanding of how God's love is revealed in Christ:

> How is that love [of God] made visible through Jesus? It is made visible in the descending way. That is the great mystery of the Incarnation.... In the gospel it's quite obvious that Jesus chose ... it not once but over and over again. At each critical moment he deliberately sought the way downwards.[2]

The closest story to the near-death experience that I can recall from my own practice involved a young adult whose cancer began when he was in high school. Tom was nineteen years old when his cancer recurred, but he refused to accept the relapse as a death sentence.

He declined further chemotherapy because there was no promise of cure even if he endured the side effects. Despite this, he still believed that he would find a way to be healed of cancer and become an "exceptional cancer patient." His parents considered taking him to court to have him declared mentally incompetent.

While he was in the hospital, the tumor advanced in his spine to the point that he was quadriplegic. Although he could neither walk nor lift his arms, he still would not believe that he was going to die from this disease. He worried whether permitting such "negative thoughts" would interfere with "positive healing thoughts."

We discharged him home in this condition on his twentieth birthday. When I visited him, he was able to move only his head and neck and required total nursing care. When we were alone, he told me of a vision that came to him while he was meditating.

Tom saw himself in a beautiful garden and saw a man there, seated on a bench. The man's fingers were like roses, and he walked with Tom in the garden and talked to him. The man touched him, and Tom reported that he moved in his bed for the first time in months. He did not want to leave the garden or the man's presence, but his companion went ahead and told him that he could not come with him yet.

I asked Tom if he knew who the man was. He said, "I *know* it was Jesus." I could tell from his eyes that he was afraid that I would not believe him: I was certain that he must be recreating the old gospel hymn "In the Garden" or were the images not the same?

I come to the garden alone,
While the dew is still on the roses.
And the voice I hear, falling on my ear,
The Son of God discloses.

And He walks with me and He talks with me,
And He tells me I am His own;
And the joy we share as we tarry there,
None other has ever known.

He speaks and the sound of His voice
Is so sweet the birds hush their singing.
And the melody that He gave to me,
Within my heart is ringing.

I'd stay in the garden with Him
Though the night around me be falling
But He bids me go, through the voice of woe,
His voice to me is calling.[3]

My question confused Tom because he had never heard of that hymn. When I sang it for him, he did not recognize the melody but responded with excitement to the parallel image to his vision that he heard in the song. Two days later, Tom told his parents that he would not live through the night, and he died peacefully in his sleep.

As I sit by the beds of these children, I have seen God's love made manifest in this descending way. I have seen Jesus Christ come repeatedly to bring peace and to link the children's stories with his own.

> They will receive from the Father a peace that the world will be powerless to destroy. It is this peace that will give new meaning to the act of believing. Now to believe will be to rejoice at Jesus' going and coming, to love him in such a way as to share his courage, to continue his mission to the same world but without coveting the world's peace.[4]

"Peace I leave with you," says Jesus. "My peace I give to you; not as the world gives do I give to you. Let not your hearts be troubled, neither let them be afraid" (John 14:27 RSV).

4

A Mystery Story

God made man because he loves stories.
ELIE WIESEL, *THE GATES OF THE FOREST*

Some people delight in turning simple truths into big mysteries. I have heard it in sermons as the preacher lingers lovingly over the very enunciation of mystery. The homiletical intention is dénouement, end of argument. *Behold, I shew you a mysssssstery!*

For medical doctors, a mystery is anything but a finale. It is more a call to action, like Teddy Roosevelt's leading the charge up San Juan Hill. How we hate unsolved mysteries!

What would you think if you had a mysterious chest pain and I said, "Ah, it's a mystery!" and walked away? So doctors and others squirm in the pew when we hear sermonizing about the mystery of suffering, focusing on the symptoms but not suggesting in any way a cause or a treatment. It is, after all, the mystery of suffering rather than a "scientific view of the world" that poses the greatest stumbling block to faith for people like me.

But the ways of children are a deep mystery. Children hold the key to unlocking life's greatest mysteries. Of all physicians, pediatricians best understand the need to live with, and even appreciate, this mystery. Always at home with the spiritual nature of children, the Great Physician was the ideal pediatrician: "O Father, Lord of Heaven and earth, I thank you for hiding these things from the clever and intelligent and for showing them to mere children" (Matthew 11:25 PHILLIPS).

When the clever are really intelligent, they look to children for answers. For our sake Jesus became a vulnerable child.

I recently consulted on an adult patient with a rare tumor. Various caregivers recorded their concerns about his mental competence, or alluded to a demanding and arrogant attitude. His original symptom was pain, and two months later that pain was only worse.

I did not find him incompetent, arrogant, or excessively demanding. But I did find him to be in pain. Despite morphine, he was in worse pain than I have ever seen any cancer patient bear. After he started treatment with chemotherapy, the morphine dose quickly diminished. Those who once thought him to be arrogant and demanding changed their opinions. His intern reported, "He's like a little kid, he's so excited about each and every improvement."

Perhaps only a pediatrician would smile in relief that a patient could earn the privilege to be seen as a child. I hope that when it is my turn to be a patient, I am equally privileged. I hope that I will have the courage to report all the mysteries that excite me.

Religious educator Sophia Cavalletti refers to a mysterious bond between God and the child. She tells of a three-year-old who grew up without religious influence and had never heard the name of God spoken. "The little one asked her father, 'Where does the world come from?' He responded with a secularized theory of the origins of the world, but added, 'However, there are those who say that all this comes from a very powerful being and they call that being God.' His daughter joyously exclaimed, 'I knew what you told me wasn't true; it is God, it is God!'"[1]

To those who care about people who suffer, the mystery can be hard to bear. It sometimes appears that God doesn't take very good care of the godly. A pastor wrote to me of his personal struggle during his seminary days:

> I worked as a chaplain . . . and was at times overwhelmed by the seeming indiscretion of suffering. Many nights I lay in bed for hours wondering if I would ever be able to inspire people to believe in God when I wasn't always sure. Rick was a teenager I got to know while I was there. He had . . . cancer and more than anything it was the courage which he demonstrated that somehow gave me strength.

In his Christmas allegory, *The Story of the Other Wise Man*, Henry Van Dyke uses holy imagination to envision a godly dream that was derailed.[2] Artaban was a fourth magi meant to join the others on their trip to Bethlehem. He was detained en route, ministering to the many unfortunates he met along the way. His life's mission seemed a failure as he lay dying in a street on Easter morning and met the risen Christ. Jesus' words to Artaban (and the parents of my patients): "Inasmuch as you have done it unto one of the least of these my brethren, ye have done it unto me" (Matthew 25:40 KJV).

One father who is a gifted storyteller wove a nightly bedtime story for his son. Ernie interrupted one story to ask,

"If I die now and you and Mom don't get to heaven for a long time, will I forget you?"

"No way, son," Dad answered. "What's a long time, anyhow? Jesus died 2000 years ago and doesn't that seem like just yesterday?"

O death where is thy sting when a loving heavenly Father coaches a human dad in the fine art of stinger-removal? A mysteriously beautiful fellowship, this fellowship of suffering.

Death stings in New Haven at my favorite vegetarian restaurant. Its walls proclaim the virtues of fiber and decry the evils of nuclear waste. They write your first name on the check at that restaurant in order to locate you when your meal is ready. Five of their waiters have spelled my name "Die" rather than "Di." Not even a famous princess came first to their minds, only their greatest fear.

I asked one young man why he thought to spell my name that way. My question made him exceedingly nervous: "I am absolutely terrified by death. I can't even tolerate to say the word." I have never had the courage to tell him that I'm an oncologist.

Eight-year-old Jason Gaes has been through surgery, chemotherapy, and radiotherapy for lymphoma, but he does not let the risk of death from "cansur" sting. If Jason could meet my frightened vegetarians, he would tell them: "Every bodys godda die sometime. If you can find it get a poster that says Help me to remember Lord that nothing is gonna happen today that you and me can't handle together. Then hang it in your room and read it at night when your scared."[3]

Oat bran and sunflower oil may reduce the risk of disease, but they will not convert the heart and cast out fear.

One particularly discouraging day at work, I tried to cheer myself up. I said to myself, *Self, what did you do today that made you feel really good?*

And I answered myself, *I spent an hour with the parents of a child who is dying.*

The fact is, some of the most peace-giving moments in my adult life have been spent with these children and their parents.

People who describe their experiences with cancer often use metaphors associated with change or conversion. One young woman without a Christian background used the term "passing from death unto life" to describe her understanding of survival of childhood Hodgkin's disease. She planned a career in medicine to fulfill her sense of being "saved for a purpose." The young people I treat for life-threatening illnesses seek a meaning in their experience.

In sharing the mystery with my patients, I find meaning for my own life. Peter Kreeft says that science only asks *what* and *how*, philosophy asks *why*, but it is religion that asks *who*.[4] God's great mystery story is, after all, a "whodunit."

Seeing, then, that we are surrounded by so great a cloud of witnesses, let us solve with patience the mystery story that is set before us.

5

Gifted Clowns

I gave this mite a gift I denied to all of you—eternal innocence. She will evoke the kindness that will keep you human. She will remind you every day that I AM WHO I AM.

MORRIS WEST, CLOWNS OF GOD

My first professional encounters with Down's syndrome were during the era when families were advised to institutionalize the mentally retarded. The medical credo of the day was that the presence of a severely retarded child disrupted family life. Pediatricians counseled parents to institutionalize "idiots" for the sake of the rest of the family.[1]

Leukemia and some other forms of cancer are more common in Down's syndrome children than in the population at large. In contrast to my other patients, years ago these special children with cancer came to us not from loving homes, but from sterile institutions. I kept asking myself how a physician can continuously subject a child to painful procedures when no one counts the quantity or quality of added days as blessed.

In the late seventies, I moved to a new position and was confronted with a refreshingly different situation. Most of my Down's patients were vibrant youngsters who lived at home in large, closely knit families. I encountered well-informed families whose retarded children knew their personal worth. These were new lessons for me to learn:

> No, it was to shame the wise that God chose what is foolish by human reckoning, and to shame what is strong that he chose what is weak by human reckoning; those whom the world thinks common and contemptible are the ones that God has chosen—those who are nothing at all to show up those who are everything. (1 Corinthians 1:27–28 PHILLIPS)

Donny's family instructed me to treat him as any other child with leukemia—just as they treated him as a normal child in all possible areas of his life. During his first admission to our hospital, I remember Donny's passionate desire not to be underestimated. I did not see the frustration and anger that I expected. I met a charming performer with years of experience playing to dense audiences of the presumably mentally able.

His parents always did their best to help Donny reach his highest potential, but there was the rest of the world to deal with. Ruth and Bob poured out their hearts to a child psychiatrist about issues surely too profound for their retarded son to comprehend. As they talked to him, Donny stood to the side, feigning disinterest. The psychiatrist noted his pretense and asked, "Donny, do people ever underestimate you?" Hand on hip, Donny shot back, "Doc, you'd better believe it!"

Donny's mother was born in Puerto Rico to a Baptist mother and a Roman Catholic father. As a child, Ruth attended services for both each Sunday, and her own approach to religion combined the best of each. Whether it be the rich symbolism of Catholicism or the Baptist emphasis on personal faith, it was very important to her that Donny's personal religious commitment be recognized. She searched for a Christian church that would allow him to learn at his own pace. When Donny's spiritual growth rate exceeded the piety pace of the "normal," she warned priests and pastors not to hold her Donny back! The retarded child I met was more thoroughly Christian than I was.

At the time of his final relapse, chemotherapy offered him no hope of long-term remission. The family planned a visit to the grandparents, who had been unable to accept this retarded grandchild. Donny climbed onto his grandmother's lap and said, "Grandma, I'm going to be with Jesus soon." His parents were astonished, since no one had taught this to him.

There are some basic flaws in the proposition that we can best apprehend spiritual truth with our most mature, most logical, most modern, and most brilliant minds. Such intellectual chauvinism is certainly in conflict with Jesus' admonition to look to the children to find the secrets of the Kingdom: "Thou hast hidden these things from the wise and understanding and revealed them to babes" (Matthew 11:25 RSV).

After Donny's death, Ruth went to work supervising the kitchen and dining room staff at the Apple Doll House restaurant, a regional program that employs adult retarded citizens. How many parents who lose a child have the privilege of going to work each day and seeing the same beloved face? Seeing Down's syndrome people each day was a miraculous way to assuage the grief and retain the wonder of the small life that was no longer part of hers. No manager could have loved her employees more than Ruth or was more gifted in affirming their worth.

One of Ruth's charges, Mary Kate, excelled as a waitress and was soon promoted to hostess. When I visited, she always served my table despite her exalted new job description. She led an active life outside of work, living in a group home with other adults with Down's syndrome and competing in a variety of sports events.

It was Christmastime when I came for lunch with three guests. While we were contemplating the excellent alternatives on the menu, Mary Kate was in the corner quietly repeating, over and over again, "Croissant, croissant, croissant." The menu was arranged by numbers to simplify things for the staff. One of my guests ordered by number, but Mary Kate was not about to have her rehearsal efforts wasted: "Would that be the ham and cheese *croissant?*"

My guest complimented her on her superb French pronunciation. Mary Kate looked down demurely and said, "Thank you, but my Spanish is so much better than my French." She and Ruth, her Spanish teacher, then treated us to a duet of "Feliz Navidad."

Speech and language do not come easily for persons with Down's syndrome and represent one of their greatest sources of frustration. It takes courage for many who are retarded to risk being understood in their native tongue, let alone a foreign language. Love like Ruth's uses imagination to fuel courage.

The most gripping description I've ever read of the prophetic role of the Down's syndrome individual is found in Morris West's novel, *Clowns of God.* West's vision of Jesus' second coming describes the returned Christ with a Down's child on his knee, serving her eucharistic bread and wine:

What better [sign] could I give than to make this little one whole and new? I could do it; but I will not. . . . I gave this mite a gift I denied to all of you—eternal innocence. . . . She will never offend me, as all of you have done. She will never pervert or destroy the works of my Father's hands. She is necessary to you. She will evoke the kindness that will keep you human. . . . She will remind you every day that I AM WHO I AM.[2]

Since the overall life expectancy for children with cancer has improved and the life-opportunities for people with Down's syndrome have advanced, more of God's prophetic clowns are with us. Each time I partake of the bread and wine, I am reminded of their kindness and the many ways they keep me human.

6

Invitation to a Feast

*May our lives be a feast: the spirit of Jesus in our midst, the
work of Jesus in our hands, the spirit of Jesus in our work.*
J. METTERNICH TEAM, "UNSER LEBEN"

Recently I breakfasted at a medium-grade diner where
I heard a man warn his son in rapid-fire Spanish that if the kid
didn't stop whining and eat his bagel, he wouldn't get to go to
McDonald's for lunch. The father had unleashed the penulti-
mate parental weapon and, by golly, it worked.

Each of us has our own concept of an ideal feast. The
feast I long for most, however, has nothing to do with choles-
terol-burdened beef and fries. Because of my acquaintance
with children with cancer, I attend more soul-fortifying
repasts than most have the opportunity to attend. May I invite
you to a feast?

At the climax of one biblical story comes a feast: "Now
Simon's mother-in-law was suffering from a high fever, and
[the disciples] asked [Jesus] about her. Then he stood over her
and rebuked the fever, and it left her. Immediately she got up
and began to serve them" (Luke 4:38–39 NRSV). The story of

healing hospitality is so important that it is included by three of the four gospel writers. I cannot read this story without thinking of Donny, my little Down's syndrome saint who taught me a great deal about the joy of servanthood.

Part of his terminal care included administering morphine through a small butterfly needle taped to the skin of his tummy. Donny smothered the small battery-operated pump that pushed the morphine with Smurf stickers. He called it his "beeper," for he was Doctor Donny, on call. For this little "doctor" with Down's syndrome, the pump anchored to his pajama waist made it possible to perfectly control his pain at home.

Hospice nurses came to adjust the dosage from time to time. Donny moved from his bedroom to the living room, where Smurf-bedecked sheets and pillowcases transformed the couch into a most acceptable base of operations. At nine years of age, he had more friends than most of us will have in longer lifetimes. At home he could visit with them in between snoozes. As the leukemia progressed, he had less energy and more catnaps.

My phone rang one evening after the nurse had visited Donny's home and told his parents that he might die that very night. His mother called to ask my opinion. When I arrived, Donny was dozing peacefully on his Smurf sofa, surrounded by friends.

Donny was paler than when I had last seen him, but his pulse was steady. "I went out of the prophecy business a long time ago," I told them. "I wish I could be sure, but you know how unpredictable these things are."

As if on cue, Donny rose from his "deathbed" with a luxuriant yawn. The Prince of Smurfs was hungry and decided to take his guests "out" to dinner. He assumed the role of *maitre d'hôtel* at a mythical restaurant and escorted us to our tables.

Invisible pad and pen poised in his hand, Donny went from guest to guest, reciting the specials of the evening. For each guest, he presented a different ethnic restaurant with a complete selection from *suppe* to *nuez*. After he took the order from his last guest (in a Mexican restaurant), he flopped back into Smurfland and resumed his nap with a self-satisfied sigh of contentment. "It won't be tonight," I confidently prophesied, and Donny grinned in his sleep.

A month later, he died. For years afterward, Ruth continued to find Smurfs in closets and drawers where he had hidden them for her to find.

To some, the gospel story of Simon Peter's mother-in-law reads as if she was healed just in time to do slave duty for the menfolk. In countless ways, my patients have been my servants. It is an irony for me that I find myself called to follow in their footsteps in an era when some women feel called to move beyond servanthood. It is precisely because Jesus, the Master of paradox, does *not* call me servant but rather, friend, that I know myself as his servant *as well as* his friend.

Tony and I first met when he was nine years old, and because of his illness, we were an important part of each other's lives for seven not-long-enough years. His life was drawing to a close as I prepared for a sabbatical year away from Yale. His parents knew that I would probably be out of the country when their son died, but we protected each other from telling Tony. The colleague who would care for him in my absence gently chided me for my cowardice.

His mom worried that I didn't know how deeply Tony felt about me, although I never really felt uninformed. He had written letters to all his brothers, but he never thought to say good-bye to me. We both assumed that we would be together for his departure from this life.

I received an invitation to his home for a dinner that Tony himself would prepare. On his next clinic visit, my patient reviewed the menu with me for the feast that he planned. He watched my eyes carefully for a hint of the respect due a chef of such competence. En route to his home for that meal, my beeper indicated an emergency page. An ambulance transported the chef to a nearby hospital with an uncontrollable seizure. The dinner was postponed.

Tony was never quite the same after that episode. Intellectually and physically he was diminished, but spiritually he was stronger. Eventually, at his home we did share a dinner of quiche and other of his favorites. After dinner, he invited me to his holy of holies to see his baseball card collection and plot my biorhythms on his computer. Several weeks later, the same computer drafted me a letter.

Tony was afraid that I did not know how he felt about me. He shared his love and his mischief in a letter that revealed all the nicknames he had for me and my colleagues. I'm glad to know he considered me "Kompetent."

My colleagues wrote to me in Germany to tell me how Tony outlived all medical expectations. At Christmas, I flew home and had the opportunity for a visit with my young friend. He was in the hospital to receive a new medication but was in good health and spirits. We faced off, bed to bedside, sizing each other up. I noticed that his hair had regrown and his face was no longer bloated from prednisone. He read my thoughts and countered, "Your hair is grayer, but you've lost weight. Do you dare to eat a quiche?"

Toward the end of our Christmas visit, both Tony and I ran out of words and nodded in farewell. As I walked out of the room to return to Germany, he said softly, "Auf wiedersehn." It would turn out that I was not there when Eastertide became his Easter time.

Lord, now let thy servant (thy served) depart in peace, according to thy word.

7

Learning a New Language

*If I speak in the tongues of mortals and of angels, but do
not have love, I am a noisy gong or a clanging cymbal.*
1 CORINTHIANS 13:1 (NRSV)

Language can be a vehicle for communication and
comfort, or, as in the case of the Tower of Babel, it can result
in confusion and alienation. Words have tremendous power
over us. For some of us, learning a new way to speak (and listen) is a requirement before we can achieve the untroubled
heart that Jesus promised.

In our fearful society, *cancer* is possibly the most dreaded
of words. During a recent hospitalization for minor surgery, I
recuperated postoperatively on the gynecological oncology floor.
My disease was neither gynecological nor malignant, but this
was the only floor of our hospital that had a bed available.

It disturbed some of my friends to find me on a cancer
ward and my nurses worried that I, too, might be upset with
my room assignment. But I was a happy patient. I value cancer nurses as the best in the profession. A psychotherapist I
know was highly agitated by this situation: "I know you keep

saying that there are worse things in life than cancer," she said, "but I sure have a hard time thinking of any. I had the same surgery a few years ago, and if I had woken up on that ward, it would have upset me a lot."

Is it possible to talk the language of cancer and have freedom from fear? Intellectual understanding about cancer does not seem to protect us against this primordial dread.

Fear is something with which we as humans are very familiar. The Bible says that fear is so typical a human response that visiting angels were careful to preface their remarks with "Be not afraid," even when they came bearing good news.

Although I may not have a heightened fear of cancer, I do know about the emotion of fear. Several years ago I had to take a medication with a peculiar side effect. I would start talking and find the thought suspended in mid-air, incomplete. I would literally have to wait for the thought to take a different path or for the lazy synapse in my brain to finally fire. It was a devastating experience. I could not do my work if I did not have quick access to words. Lives depend on the quick firing of my brain. Never in my life have I been more depressed or more afraid. I remember praying at the time, "Lord, take my life but don't touch one neuron of my beautiful brain."

As soon as the prayer was launched, I realized its folly. It was painful to realize that my adult relationship with God was grounded in intellectual apprehension, a half-brained spirituality. I may have given lip service to the spiritual gifts of the retarded, but was I really ready to be equal with someone like Donny?

I was not the only one whose life was influenced by Donny. Roger's personal struggle with cancer was a particularly difficult one. This teenager endured chemotherapy impatiently and with great anguish. When the first program failed to cure him, he faced more rigorous treatment. He was unwilling to talk about it and unable to find meaning in his own predicament.

Roger's friends had trouble in their attempts to help him until a high school classmate invited him to training sessions for the Special Olympics. He met Donny at the local center for the retarded and handicapped and was caught up by the infectious love of all the Down's syndrome children who reached out and touched him. He volunteered to accompany them to the state Special Olympics.

Roger approached his treatment the next week quite differently. With chemotherapy running in a vein but displaying a radiant face, he asked me, "Do you know I went to the Special Olympics and met Donny? It changed my life!"

Some of us are quick with our tongues, yet others find our tongues a natural hindrance. Artie was Tom's brother. Tom, you will remember, died in his bedroom shortly after he had a vision of Jesus visiting him in a garden. Tom had shared the dream with his Down's syndrome brother, Artie.

The morning of Tom's death Artie had nothing to say. He packed his books and went to the curb to wait for the school bus as he always did. His parents wondered how, in his simplicity, he had processed that loss. It was as though nothing unusual had happened in his life that day.

In the months that followed Tom's death, Artie was consumed with his own activities, preparing for the winter competition of the Special Olympics. Artie's performance was truly amazing, the ski champion's neck bowing under the many medals. Bursting with pride, he joined the other athletes for a press conference.

"This has been a very exciting day, Artie," said the sportscaster. "What were you thinking about when you crossed the finish line?"

Ordinarily, Artie's speech is very difficult to understand, but his response was clearly heard: "My brother died this year."

"I'm sure he was an inspiration to you," replied the stunned sportscaster.

"Yes!" answered Artie.

Wolf Wolfensberger calls this phenomenon "speaking in tongues"—a person whose ordinary speech is unintelligible suddenly speaks clearly, revealing an important truth.[1] Sometimes, modern technology helps in the interpretation of those tongues. Linguists in California find that the keyboard of a computer can free some Down's syndrome children with faulty speech to express themselves quite poetically. A teenager named Christine chose to write about God and turned to the researcher to say, "He's gonna like this." I am sure she is right. She wrote, "I like God's finest whispers."[2]

A children's hospital is a school for fine whispers where most of the students are parents. A mother in Wisconsin whose eight-year-old daughter died twenty-five years ago wrote to tell me what she learned:

> Many times we said that we thought she was a little missionary sent from God. We, her family, have been taught so much through her. Becky told us that she had the most wonderful prayer in her heart to God. A little later she said, "Do you know what God said to me in my heart? He said, 'Yea, though ye walk through the valley of the shadow of death, ye shall fear no evil.'" Then she added, "Nothing could break the chain from my heart to God's heart—nothing in the world."

Donny's family teaches me that the origin of prayer is in the soul, not in the head. During a hospitalization for a blood-borne infection, his parents lamented his terminal condition and their lack of preparedness for his death. "We don't want him to suffer, but we are not ready for him to die. We pray that God will not take him yet."

Several days later, we sent him home without further treatment. Without antibiotics his fever resolved; and without chemotherapy his leukemic cells were replaced by normal white blood cells capable of fighting infection. This "spontaneous" remission lasted long enough for him to die at home many months later surrounded by family and his many friends.

Before the diagnosis of cancer, many of my patients and their parents do not have much experience in listening for these whispers. Tony and his family attended church regularly, but prayer became a new language for him when his leukemia advanced to his brain as well as his bone marrow. It was time to prepare his family for the inevitable. Along with the medical details of clinical death, I mentioned the religious experiences that other families have described.

Tony recovered from this particular episode, but some weeks later, his mother reported that, out of the blue, Tony said, "He wants me."

His mother was frightened but found the courage to ask, "Do you mean God?"

When he answered affirmatively, his mother asked him if God spoke to him in a dream.

"No. He speaks to me when I pray."

"What do you mean, when you pray?"

"I start praying, and then I listen."

"Is it scary?"

"No. It's peaceful."

A frightened mother chose just to listen. Some weeks later, he said, "I don't want to die yet. Gerry is only three and is not old enough to understand. I've been able to talk to each of my other brothers to prepare them, and they'll be okay. I can leave a letter for Gerry, but it's not the same. If I could live just one more year, I could explain it to him myself, and he would understand. Three is just too young."

I explained to the mother that it was just not medically possible for him to survive that additional year. Tony lived for exactly one year after that honorable prayer.

Sometimes a new language is learned through dreams. One of my patients was a three-month-old baby boy who was admitted to the hospital with a cancer that began in the adrenal gland and now spread to the liver. I had few encouraging words as I made rounds. My heart went out to Naomi, the young mother who sat at her firstborn's cribside.

"Do you believe in healing?" she asked. That seemed to me a strange question to pose to a doctor she didn't know. I asked her to tell me something about herself.

Naomi and her husband were raised in a mainline Protestant church and had not returned since their wedding. Their early married life was full and happy, but their baby's desperate situation now made her ask whether something important was missing.

Naomi knew a woman whose life was changed by a charismatic renewal experience. This woman often retreated into a room in her home that she had converted into a shrine for healing prayer. At the same time she grew increasingly alienated from her husband, who did not share these beliefs and practices. In her time of crisis, Naomi wanted to seek all possible alternatives that might help her child, but she was frightened that such a search might damage her marriage as it had her friend's.

I shared with Naomi some of the struggles that others have faced with that question. I told her that I hoped that if she prayed for her son to be healed, she would also be willing to ask her husband to join her to put their lives in God's hands, whether little Henry lived or not.

That weekend, she and Jim, her husband, asked a hospital chaplain to baptize the baby and pray for his healing. On Monday, Henry was a little better, but Naomi's appearance was transformed. She told me of the events of the weekend and said, "I don't know if Henry will be healed, but I feel as if I've been healed."

When the baby did not survive, I wondered how one could "find God" while hoping for healing and yet stay faithful after that hope had vanished. Several years later, Naomi wrote to me to tell me of a dream she had.

Naomi dreamed that she and the baby were in the kitchen of the church where she grew up. Henry was crawling around on the floor, and every time he got to a certain place in the center, he'd say, "God!" He was very happy, like a child greeting a well-known and trusted friend—or parent.

In her dream, Naomi commented to a friend, who was also in the church kitchen, that it gave her goosebumps. It was as though Henry could see God, although she and her friend could not. Then, the next time he reached the center, Henry died. His legs buckled under him, and he threw his head back to look at her once more and reached out an arm. Naomi rushed over to him and grabbed his hand, but it was too late. His eyes were blank. Her baby was dead.

"Suddenly," Naomi described, "God strode in and scooped up my little one and perched him on his arm. Henry sat on God's arm with a hand on God's shoulder, laughing and chattering with him." Naomi could see that the baby was fine and happy and that he knew God well, but she was sad that she could not hold him anymore. "God saw how sad I was and felt sorry for me, and so he handed Henry to me and said I could keep him for a while longer until my baby returned from the mission he had before him. Henry was fine now, although not as animated with me as I held him. It was as though my child had been handed from a Parent to a trusted baby-sitter." He was in her arms but watching God.

As God was leaving, Naomi asked, "Will I have other children I can keep?" She goes on, "God stopped and looked at me with so much love, it was overwhelming. He said gently, in a way that made me feel especially cared for, 'Everyone's life has a plan.'" Naomi held Henry's cheek to her own and tried to figure out whether God's look had betrayed any sorrow (that she would not get her wish) or amusement (that good things were ahead for her). "But there was neither, just love, overwhelming love. That was what mattered and that was what the answer was—not yes or no, but God's love."

In the years since the baby's death, Naomi and Jim became the proud parents of two healthy babies. Perhaps it's an occupational hazard, but since this mysterious dream-prayer was first shared with me, I have tried many times to *analyze* it. While my attempts to understand the dream have always fallen short, each time I have *told* her story, some say that they, like Naomi, were "healed."

One of the Greek words in the New Testament for healing implies salvation. Spiritual healing does not restore a person to the place they were before the illness. It provides a more comprehensive health-care package. The peace and healing of God that defies human understanding can bring us salvation and keep our hearts and minds untroubled—even when they do not satisfy our analytical inclinations!

8

Angels and Other Strangers

~~~❦~~~

Do not neglect to show hospitality to strangers, for by doing
that some have entertained angels without knowing it.
HEBREWS 13:2 (NRSV)

I've spoken with many who are skeptical about the so-called "near-death experiences" of adults. They claim that many of these phenomena are culturally determined and reflect the background of the individual. Similar opinions have been used to minimize the importance of the spiritual comments of children facing death.

I had a phone call from a journalist who was following up on a wire-service report of my work with terminally ill children. "Did any of the children say what Jesus looked like?" he asked.

I am not sure what he thought of my response: "You know, the children weren't exactly sitting there with pen and pad poised to take notes in case they later ran into a skeptical adult. The only story I can tell you is what he *doesn't* look like."

I once heard a story of a young child who was not ill but died quite unexpectedly in an accident. On an occasion prior to her death, she looked up at an artist's rendition of Jesus and said emphatically, "He doesn't look like that at all!"

This child's story is not unique. It manifests the remarkable ability of children to express their own spiritual gifts, despite what adults have to say.

When Ann married, she gave up her nominal Christian belief since it seemed irrelevant to her new life. Although she and her husband enjoyed economic privilege, romance faded early and she soon considered her marriage a disaster. But their lifestyle, including a new mink coat, had its rewards.

Ann adored her youngest son, T. J. She told a friend, once, that if anything happened to this marvelous five-year-old, they would have to lock her up. Ann never sent the children to Sunday school, and the name of God was never mentioned in their house.

One day T. J. said out of the blue, "Mama, I love you more than *anything* in the world, except God. And I love him a little bit more!" Ann was taken aback and told him that this was okay as long as it was God he loved more than her. *But why would T. J. speak of God?* she pondered. Even more mysterious was why he should love a God whose name he had never heard from her lips.

Two days later they suffered one of the coldest days of an already bitterly cold winter. While T. J.'s sister was horseback riding, the little boy crossed a snow-covered creek and broke through the ice. He must have died immediately, although it took the family an hour and a half to find him. The first words out of Ann's mouth when she heard the news were, "I hate you, God!"

Even as she spit out the words, Ann felt herself held in loving arms. Can you truly hate someone whom you have never in some way loved?

As her world shattered around her, she remembered another mysterious thing that T. J. had done that week. He had purchased a Christmas gift for her at the Secret Santa shop at school and kept trying to give it to her before Christmas. Each time he tried to give it to her, she laughed and told him to put it away until Christmas. He was persistent, but his mother prevailed.

When Ann got home from the stables where T. J. died, she ran upstairs to the place he had hidden it. She opened the box to find a beautiful necklace with a cross.

As Ann looks back now, she says that Jesus dealt with her the way a loving parent deals with a hurt child. "He made me reach out to others rather than get lost in myself. Helping others helped me." Prior to the accident, Ann's husband had no religious belief, but he was the first to cry out to God for help and sensed an immediate response to his prayer. Slowly, their old materialistic lives melted away, their marriage healed, and they described themselves as new creatures in Christ.

Through her ordeal, Ann discovered she had a gift of spiritual hospitality, bringing healing to other parents. Henri Nouwen characterizes healing as a form of hospitality:

> Healing means, first of all, the creation of an empty but friendly space where those who suffer can tell their story to someone who can listen with real attention. Healers are hosts who patiently and carefully listen to the story of the suffering stranger. Patients are guests who rediscover their selves by telling their story to the one who offers them a place to stay.[1]

This young mother has reached out to over 200 families whose children suffered accidental deaths. In sharing her own story, Ann has learned that many parents felt that their children knew they were going to die. She calls her effort "T. J. Ministries," not only after her T. J., but to emphasize how she has made it since then—*Through Jesus.*

Not all strangers are unknown to each other. Some become strangers to each other through the painful process of failed marriage, followed by divorce. In my practice, this represents one of the most difficult situations in the care of a child.

There is an enormous additional burden when family strife accompanies the seriously ill child to the hospital. Because of divorce and remarriage, my young patient Bill had four parents. Bill's prayer was for them to be one family, with one heart and a new spirit.

At the time he was diagnosed with leukemia, Bill's biological parents and stepparents thought they were doing their best to survive divorce, remarriage, and the sharing of children. What helped them most was living far away from each other and limiting their social intercourse to small-talk at drop-off and pick-up exchanges of the children. They were more successful than most families in similar situations, and Bill certainly did not seem damaged by belonging to a less-than-old-fashioned American family unit. In fact, it was in the context of the reorganized family that he began to think about God.

The initial contact of the quartet of parents in the hospital was highly civil. When the stress of former spouses in daily contact finally hit, this group did the unprecedented. They knew the source of their tension, and rather than displacing their family anger onto the medical staff, they talked to each other. It shocked Kathy to realize that she had more in common with her ex-husband's new wife than with any other woman in her acquaintance. The mother and stepmother formed a nucleus for reconciliation and communication.

When Bill relapsed and his death appeared inevitable, he indicated a desire to die at home. In attempting to honor that request, we found that it would not be medically easy. He came to our hospital from a distant region that had no type of hospice care to offer at home. With the help of a nurse who lived in their community, the four parents lived under the same roof, sharing the nursing responsibilities. After Bill died, they invited me to dinner.

The house looked like a new home when I drove up. During the final weeks of Bill's illness, the two fathers had made significant progress on home repairs. The two mothers worked together in the kitchen on the meal. The four of them had shopped together to buy me a gift. Now they spoke of their future plans.

The Christmas holidays loomed ahead. No other friends or family members could really understand the anticipated emptiness of the season to come. Bill's birthday was near Christmas, and the festivities for all of them had become irrevocably tied to that event. They planned to spend all the holidays from Thanksgiving through the New Year as an extended family. Through Bill and in Christ, they had been reconciled.

In human terms, the battle lines of truth and evil seem never more easily drawn than in a failing marriage and divorce. In each such personal "holy war" for truth, the enemy seems only too clear to envision. Yet Christian philosopher Richard Mouw warns us that

The only two actors in the cosmic drama whose performances [for good and evil] we can count on are God and Satan. Once we get to the level of human performance, the lines are more difficult to draw. . . . We will often misidentify truths and errors if we think in rigid "us versus them" categories. We would do well to exercise caution in how we draw the battle lines.[2]

Child psychiatrist Albert Solnit knows that he is not using paradigms of the judicial system when he speaks about divorce. He suggests that divorced parents should apply the wisdom of Solomon and the Golden Rule rather than to look out for their own interests in child custody.[3] Solnit points out that the court too often looks to the interests of the adults and wields the knife over the child to satisfy the parents, even when it would fatally divide the child.

Philosopher Mouw's and psychiatrist Solnit's words are wise, albeit seemingly impossible in terms of human understanding. And yet, we are promised that the wolf shall dwell with the lamb. The prophet Isaiah also says that in that day of the humanly impossible, a little child shall lead them.

9

Does Jesus Drive
a School Bus?

Children have to be educated but they also have to be
left to educate themselves.

ERNEST DIMNET, *THE ART OF THINKING*

The parents of an eight-year-old boy with cancer
avoided discussing his impending death from cancer or matters of faith despite obvious signs that their son would die
within a few days. The boy took them by surprise one morning with the report of a dream.

In the dream a big yellow school bus pulled up to his
house and the door opened. On the bus he saw Jesus, who told
him of his impending death and invited him to go with him
on the bus. In his dream, he accepted Jesus' invitation. It was
with great peace that he recounted this dream to his parents.

Of all of the images I've heard from children, the
school bus has become my favorite. So I was puzzled when I
told this story to child psychiatrist Kyle Pruett and watched
his brow furrow solemnly. Was there a psychoanalytical

interpretation at variance with the Christian message I read into the dream? Instead, he narrated the significance of the school bus from a loving father's point of view.

Several weeks before our conversation, the entire Pruett family drove the eldest daughter to begin her college career in a distant state. As they neared their destination, Kyle was confronted by a memory from his daughter's childhood that returned to him unbidden. "We were at the curb on her first day of kindergarten, and I could see that big, old yellow school bus pull up. I could even see, hear, and feel that huge door *slam* in my face, taking my daughter away from me. I had completely forgotten how wrenching an experience that was for me—not at all nice!"

At a nursery school where Dr. Pruett consults, the model of a yellow school bus is worn out and requires replacement faster than any other toy. In playing with the bus, these youngsters master separation from their parents.

If children must master separation from their parents, the converse must also be true: Parents must master separation from their children. But this presupposes an earlier step. Ethicist William May reminds us that the first task of parenthood is to master *attachment* to the "little stranger."[1] May warns us that the baby's arrival upsets the myth that a child will extend the familiar. Instead, it pushes the parents into the novel and strange.

On the same wards of my own hospital where parents mourn the loss of the children from cancer, we mourn the fact that today too few parents master attachment to their children. In the same medical center where we miraculously rejuvenate lungs, livers, and bone marrows, we cannot seem to save enough children who are sickened by social despair.

A colleague, who works in behavioral pediatrics, commented to me, "The children's psychiatric ward is really getting me down. Isn't it ironic that I come to talk to you, an *oncologist*, to cheer up? Tell me some of your stories about your patients. I want to feel good. What kind of crazy world is this?"

Part of the craziness in the world are the rules that some physicians make to distance themselves from patients. A colleague hesitated to write to a family when their daughter came to mind a year after her death. He was concerned that contact from the medical staff would make the family sad and invade their privacy. He shared this concern some time later at an informal meeting of our staff with the child's father. "What's the worst thing that could happen to me?" smiled this big ex-football player. "I might cry? Big deal!"

A young physician commented that he had read in a textbook that it was pathological for grieving to extend more than a year after the death. The dad's eyes gleamed moistly, "Do you really think that a day goes by that I *don't* think about her? That doesn't mean that life doesn't go on or I am unable to function. How could I *ever* forget her?"

Another father whose professional field is communication used his computer to compose dialogue with his son about daily family life and how he feels in the years following the young man's death. A mother whose child died seven years ago cannot trim a Christmas tree without thinking of her son standing by her side, backseat driving the placement of each ornament. "Can a mother forget her child?" analogizes the God who promises never to forget us.

I recently met a young couple who lost identical twins to the same disease. Nathan and Jordan loved school buses and would ask every visitor to their home to draw a school bus with Jesus, their parents and grandparents, and them aboard. Nate was never able to walk and died at three years of age, three months before his brother, Jordan.

Shortly before Nate's death, the entire family went on a trip on a school bus that turned out to be a disaster. The driver went too fast over a pothole, and they were all roughly thrown around. Little Nate was thrown into the aisle, and his mom caught him just in time to prevent serious injury. This upset the twins very much and made it very important for them to know who drove a school bus. Dr. Pruett recalls the same preoccupation of his daughters. At the dinner table, the family would often hear the comparative merits (and demerits) of the current driver. It mattered very much who was in control of that school bus.

Although they knew that they would lose the second little guy, these young parents bravely attempted to answer Jordan's questions about death, heaven, and his brother. They were never able to begin the process of grieving for Nathan as long as they faced the unfinished business of Jordan's impending death. Remembering the rough ride in the bus, Jordan commented, "Nate with Jesus. Nate no more owies."

A few days after Nathan's funeral, Jordan asked his aunt, "What Nate doing?"

Auntie stretched her imagination to paint a picture for him: "Well, I bet Nate's running in the grass with Jesus, with no shoes on!"

"Silly Nate!" exclaimed his brother as he laughed and gazed upward, as if to see Nate, who could not even walk in his lifetime, running with Jesus.

This became his favorite image of heaven, and when he went for a walk, he would insist on walking through the tall grass at the side of the road. A month later, he told his grandmother, "Oma, Nate's running through the grass with Jesus. Nate no shoes on. Nate all better."

The parents choked back their tears each time Jordan would ask to go pick Nathan up to bring him home. Whenever he asked to go to see his brother in heaven, he accepted their answer of, "Soon, Jordan, you will go to see Jesus and Nathan in heaven."

One day he became very thoughtful for a moment, thinking of his brother and how he would get to heaven to join him. He asked, "Dad, does Jesus drive a school bus?"

10

Surviving the Holocaust

~~~~~~~~

*Has all this suffering, this dying around us, a meaning?
For, if not, then ultimately there is no meaning to survival; for a life whose meaning depends upon such a
happenstance—as whether one escapes or not—ultimately would not be worth living at all.*

VIKTOR FRANKL, MAN'S SEARCH FOR MEANING

I would like to end this book with the previous chapter,
to simply witness that God is alive, interested, and loving. I would
like to say amen with the children safe in the arms of Jesus.

A parent recently reminded me that belief can be a
more painful proposition than unbelief. The unbeliever
assumes that no One is responsible or holds an answer. Belief
to these parents suggests that there is some One who holds all
answers. For every young heart untroubled, there may be one
or more older hearts left unsure.

A year before Tony died, I had to give him a spinal
treatment. My beloved young friend choked back his tears as
he entered the treatment room although we both knew he
would cooperate. The dirty deed would be done with no dis-

cussion, without a struggle. I had feelings of anger and frustration that day, and my feelings poured upward: "Don't You care at all?"

I personally hold that there is no pain on this earth to compare with the loss of a child. If there is such a thing as the survival of the fittest, the fit surely do not seem very fit to accept their survival. For every holocaust, there is a variation on the "survivors' syndrome."

When I was a medical student, I participated in the interview of a patient admitted to a psychiatric hospital for depression. The patient was a Jew who had survived Hitler's "final solution." His young daughter did not survive, however, and he could not forget the day that decided her fate. The guards paraded the inmates before them to decide who would be chosen for slave labor and who would be used for "medical experimentation." This man walked hand in hand with his daughter as they approached the guard.

The guard indicated that the father should join the labor force to the left, but his daughter should go with the group to the right. As they understood the implication, his daughter held his hand tighter and begged her papa to protect her. The impatient soldier poised his bayonet over their clutched hands in unambiguous threat. As the child grasped her father's hand the tighter, the guard suddenly lowered the bayonet and this poor man let go of his daughter's hand. She was led away to the right and to her death. The father survived but was haunted for the rest of his life by the fact that he had let go of her hand. He saw her death as his own fault.

There are countless ways a parent can perceive that he or she has let go of the child's hand. A mother called me a few years ago to tell me a story and ask me a question. Her son was three years old when he developed cancer. Despite multiple relapses and threat of death many times, he did survive. His potential mortality from cancer was no longer an issue.

What this mom wished to share were the circumstances surrounding her son's conception. If there was a way for her to turn back the clock, she never would have attempted to abort her pregnancy. She was not married to the child's father and he did not want this child. He offered her a medication with the intention to terminate her pregnancy. When the pregnancy was not aborted, he threw her out.

Her question to me many years later was, "Do you think that the concoction I drank caused the cancer?"

I told her that we will never know what caused the cancer, but that it was not possible to live so many years with that memory without suffering from the burden. She later wrote that although her own religious tradition preached forgiveness through acceptance of Christ's sacrifice, she had never been able to forgive herself and had rejected the forgiveness that God offered in Jesus.

She felt there was no one in her church with whom she could share this burden. Most would have been shocked that she had been so sinful. Others might have advised her that it was her choice, not a reason for guilt. After "confessing" to me, she underlined every passage in her Bible that referred to God's forgiveness. She was amazed that the burden was finally lifted. She had finally forgiven herself. The healing of memories can be more difficult to accomplish than the healing of cancer. Her son has been in remission and presumably cured for several decades.

I have watched over the years to observe, not which Scripture passages are recommended to these parents by their pastors, but what parts of the Bible they seek on their own. There are three passages that they study and restudy: Jesus in the Garden of Gethsemane, the story of Job, and the story of Abraham and Isaac on Mount Moriah. Death-camp survivor and historian Elie Wiesel reminds us that Abraham was asked on the mount, literally, to bring the only son he loved and to bind him to the altar in a holocaust.

It is my observation that parents tend to see their child's illness most often in terms of their own failure. In fact, when I am asked, "Do you know why children get cancer?" I always assume the real question is, "What did *I* do wrong that *my* child got cancer?"

Wiesel tells us that one unusual Midrashic (Jewish commentary on the Scripture) explanation of the *Akeda* (Hebrew name for the story of Mount Moriah) attributes God's challenge to Abraham as punishment for his rejection of his other son, Ishmael.[1]

What was father Abraham thinking on the way up the mount? Where did he find the courage to take the first step toward what was promised to be a horrible death of his beloved son and his own dreams? Psychiatrist and Holocaust survivor Viktor Frankl tells of an old Viennese saying that he used in counseling fearful patients: It is better to have a horrible ending than to experience horror without ending.[2] Faith would rather take the first step toward what would seem to be a holocaust than live through a thousand imaginary holocausts without end. Father Abraham was put to a test of faith in the face of a holocaust and so was son Viktor.

As the Nazi nightmare continued to ravage Austria and countless Jews were deported from Vienna, Viktor Frankl waited for his visa to emigrate to the United States before it was too late. He feared, however, what would happen to his elderly parents if he were to leave. The day the coveted visa arrived, the burden of his parents' potential fate lay heavily on his heart. He covered the yellow *Judenstern* on his jacket lapel with his briefcase and entered Stephansdom, Vienna's main cathedral, in time for the Wednesday concert. As the organist played, Frankl wrestled in his soul.

He arrived home to find his father excited about a piece of marble that he held in his hands. On his walk that day, his father passed by the destroyed synagogue and found this broken piece. It was a part of the sacred law, a fragment of eternal truth rescued from the hideous rubble of National Socialism. Father and son looked together to see which of the commandments it represented. The single Hebrew letter gave the clue: "Honor thy father and thy mother that thy days may be long upon the land."[3]

In the Old Testament, father Abraham had the outrageous faith to believe that God would honor his promise to make him the father of many nations. In another era, son Viktor had the courage to give up his visa to certain freedom. He remained in the Nazi-occupied land with his vulnerable parents. He was able to protect them for several more years. He went with them to the camps where both his mother and father met their deaths. Frankl survived to tell his patients and the world about self-sacrificing love. God's law and its promises were written on his heart.

And my own Mount Moriah looms on the horizon.

11

Facing Mount Moriah

❦

Abraham took the wood of the burnt offering and laid it on his son Isaac and he himself carried the fire and the knife. So the two of them walked on together.

GENESIS 22:6 (NRSV)

Abraham hears a Voice say, "I am the Lord, thy God. Thou shalt have no other gods before me."

"By all means, Lord," he replies with pious courtesy. "The new BMW, a fancier house, a summer cottage on the beach—they mean nothing to me anymore. I've learned my lesson. I denounce keeping up with the Joneses."

"Abraham!" comes the Voice, now louder. "Thou shalt have no other gods before me!"

"I heard you, Lord. Believe me, I have denounced my workaholic ways. Nothing is more important to me than my family. I denounce any worldly ambitions that would separate me from my family. I place power, ambition, riches, and fame all on the altar. You have gotten your point across. Trust me."

"Abraham, Abraham! Thou shalt have no other gods before me!"

Many of the parents I meet start their journeys thinking that this is the answer. They used to live shallow, materialistic lives, and they now hear God saying that there is something better for them. For many fathers, work has alienated them from their wives and children, and so they naturally assume that God's message is simply to invest more time in their families. Certainly this is a healthy part of the message, but few suspect that it is not the whole story.

"For God's sake, I'm getting a headache!" complains Abraham. "What other gods could you possibly mean? I've covered a lot of territory in my time and heard about a lot of so-called gods but none of those pathetic idols can compare to you, Yahweh! Besides, you and I have a covenant."

"Ah, the covenant, Abraham. Do you love me more than the covenant?"

"What are you talking about, Yahweh? Of course I do. A covenant is a concept. You are the Living God."

"The covenant is through your seed Isaac. Abraham, do you love me more than Isaac?"

Abraham turns pale. Isaac senses his dis-ease and grasps his papa's hand tightly.

Jesus restated it this way: "Whoever comes to me and does not hate father and mother, wife and children, brothers and sisters, yes, and even life itself, cannot be my disciple" (Luke 14:26 NRSV).

"Hate my child?" thunders Abraham. *"What are you talking about, God? Have you forgotten what Isaac was all about? He's the seed for the covenant. Without my child, you have no covenant, no people, no future on this meshugah planet.*

"You're changing the rules, Yahweh," he continues. *"Have you heard the joke going around the Jewish community since the Holocaust, Yahweh? 'Chosen people,' uh? Next time, choose somebody else."*

"Abraham, Abraham, Abraham! Thou shalt have no other gods before me!"

For some of us who have not given life to another human being, our lives may still bear fruit that is at risk of becoming an idol. I ask myself who or what my own Isaac is, as I sit at the computer at two in the morning lovingly shaping and rewriting this manuscript.

"Di, do you hate the book for my sake?"

"What are you talking about, Lord? Isn't the book your work?"

"Which do you love more, Di, the God of Abraham, Isaac, and Jacob or your book about the God of Abraham, Isaac, and Jacob?"

The problem with holocausts is that we learn that even the professed believer may worship a graven image that barely resembles the Creator, Redeemer, and Sustainer of the universe.

Viktor Frankl went to Auschwitz with the pages of a manuscript secreted in his coat, only to be forced to part with the garment once he arrived. He describes his grieving for the loss of that work: "Thus I had to undergo and to overcome the loss of my mental child. And now it seemed as if nothing and no one would survive me; neither a physical nor mental child of my own!"[1]

Instead of his own coat with the hidden book, he inherited the tattered rags of someone who was sent directly to the gas chamber on arrival. Coincidence is not a term that he would choose to accept for what he discovered in the pocket of this garment: "Instead of the many pages of my manuscript, I found in a pocket of the newly acquired coat one single page torn out of a Hebrew prayer book, containing the most important Jewish prayer, *Shema Yisrael*." (Found in Deuteronomy 6:4–5, the prayer reads, "Hear, O Israel: The LORD is our God, the LORD alone. You shall love the LORD your God with all your heart, and with all your soul, and with all your might" [NRSV].)

A colleague came to my office, troubled about the mother of one of his patients. "She's lost her faith," he worries. "She prayed that the child would be healed. Now she is angry at God."

A nurse expressed concern about a father who sits in his son's room rereading the same passages of the Bible that he had claimed in faith that his son would be healed. Now he is frightened and angry, but he keeps reading all the same.

These parents may be angry enough to "hate" God, but they have not lost their belief. True atheists should be at peace with their conclusion, not restlessly angry at the Nonexistent and everyone who does believe. They have not lost the true God but simply come to the brokenness of the truly spiritual person who must resign from trying to be God for their loved ones. During the dark night of the soul, they are angry at the world's most patient Lover.

As helpful as our own families may be, as constrained as we may be to honor them, on Mount Moriah we are like orphaned children, on our own. It is on Moriah that we learn that our parents, our traditions, our culture have added jots and tittles to the law. The first commandment remains simple, to have no other gods before God. Our task on Moriah is to learn what this means in our own families, in our own times, and in our own traditions. On Moriah we are alone with God.

Old Testament theologian Phyllis Trible believes Abraham's faith was challenged because of his idolatry of his son. Abraham had allowed Isaac to replace Yahweh as the primary object of his adoration. She sees the resolution of Abraham's test as an experience of healing:

> In adoring Isaac, Abraham turns from God. The test, then, is an opportunity for understanding and healing. To relinquish attachment is to discover a glorious freedom. To give up human anxiety is to receive divine assurance. To disavow idolatry is to find God.[2]

Abraham was not Isaac's only parent, and Trible is not the only contemporary theologian to complain that the biblical story of Mount Moriah has omitted an important woman. We are left to imagine what Isaac's mother, Sarah, thought of the whole process. Did she even know what Abraham was up to that day? Trible regrets for Sarah that the mother who idolized the boy was not permitted to participate in the healing.

Some women who were the victims of incest or child abuse at the hands of their fathers suggest that no mother would ever take her child up that mountain as father Abraham did. Yet every day in my clinic, I watch *Sarahs* lead their tearful children to the treatment room and hope that the first Sarah's good fortune will parallel their own. I know many mothers as well as fathers who have memorized the craggy rocks of Moriah's topography.

I have heard the stories of many fathers who, in the moment of their child's own suffering, have been haunted by memories of the civilians they killed as soldiers in Vietnam. These men have come to mistrust their ability under pressure to be fully human for another human being. As often as I have heard about the My Lai massacre from fathers of that generation, I have also heard about contemplated or attempted abortions of this particular child's pregnancy from mothers. Other parents' stories may be less dramatic, but each *Sarah* and each *Abraham* bring the pages of their own human history to the base of that awful mountain as they ask, "Why me?" It is only the children on Moriah whose list of regrets makes short reading.

Psychiatrist Scott Peck, who participated in the investigations of My Lai during the Vietnam War, warns that the tendency to avoid pain and suffering is "the primary basis of all human mental illness."[3] Perhaps this is why I can recall so many parents who have experienced unbelievable holocaust through loving a child with cancer but seem so mentally healthy.

I once shared Peck's unusual definition with a pediatrician who is the son of an esteemed Orthodox Jewish scholar. He brooded for a moment, then reflected, "That's not a medical concept; that's a theological point of view."

God called out, "Abraham!" and the patriarch answered, "Here I am." We do not know Sarah's version of the story, but we do know about one of her descendants, generations later. When God's angel Gabriel called to an unwed pregnant teenager, Mary answered, like Abraham, "Here am I." In a recent talk to hospice volunteers, I reached for a suitable metaphor to impart something of the beauty of the mothers with whom I work. *I have met Mary many times.*

Time after time, I see young mothers who keep strange things and ponder them in their hearts, mystified women whose precocious children seem preoccupied with their Father's business. And yes, also the pietà—like Mary, they cradle the broken body of a great little miracle as they once had held a newborn in swaddling clothes. I have met Marys with many faces and marvel at their serenity and courage. Sarah's son survived, but Mary's Son became the lamb that God provided. *You've suffered much, Mary, and you walked back down Calvary's hill alone, without your Son. But truly you are blessed amongst women. Through you, Sarah receives her healing.*

It is another one of those gray days when I must set out for Moriah to meet my newest Sarah and Abraham and Isaac. I have set up a base camp at the foot of the mountain because I must return so often. There is a nice big rock at my camp that has become "my rock." The peak of the mount is wrapped in mist tonight, and there is an ominous wind starting to make its presence felt as I set myself down on my rock, looking up.

Moriah is not only treacherous but ugly. A few hundred yards ahead I see the bare reminder of the trail that was last pursued to the top. I have never seen undergrowth spring back as fast as on Moriah, making it more difficult for newcomers to find the previously blazed trail. The vegetation on Moriah seems to have germinated in Hades, implanting itself as mature brush when the winds blow it in. The thorn bushes here do not even bother with the mockery of berries. No one who comes here would be fooled anyway, and none can escape the nasty encounter by choosing an easier path.

Some other Abrahams and Sarahs and even Isaacs have come back from the peak to write their own trail guides. Some of them speak of the literary process as exorcism. You would have to share in a Moriah experience to fully understand the metaphor.

These volumes line the shelves of my office and are well-worn by pilgrims, but they seem almost useless the night before the journey. The ink seems temporarily to fade on the pages, as if to lower its voice to a respectful whisper.

I don't like the feel of the wind on my face tonight as I look to the distance for the little family. It is Abraham I see first, simply because the former marine is so tall and powerfully built that he cannot be missed. Ordinarily people smile ironically when they see him dwarf the tiny slip of a girl they call Sarah who is walking at his side. Child of a farm, Sarah's diminutive size disguises her strength.

As they come closer, I can see that although Abraham is carrying the supplies, it is Sarah who bears Isaac in her arms. She carried him for nine months in her body, and there is no way to prevent her from carrying him now. The child has not been able to walk for many months and despite his bulk, she carries him effortlessly.

A long time ago I indicated to her my amazement at her physical strength. She laughed and retorted that her daddy told her that if she picked up a calf on the day it was born and every day thereafter, by the time the beast was full grown, she might even be able to pick up the whole cow. I was never one to argue with the earthy wisdom of farmers.

Mother and father put down their burdens temporarily, and we plan the strategy for the ascent. Abraham puts his arm around Sarah tenderly to shield her from the frightful wind, and I imagine that I see their entire history as lovers flash in his eyes. In a single moment, he recalls and regrets each time he has treated her shabbily and undervalued one of the most admirable human beings he (and I) will ever be privileged to know. The intensity of his love is mirrored there as well. We have been through too much together for me to turn my eyes away as an embarrassed voyeur.

They understand that I can go no further with them. In our months and years together, I have only been able to train them in the tactics of a Moriah climb. The trail guide must remain below when the *trek is finally made. I wait until Sarah has Isaac safely snuggled in her arms before I embrace them both. Her eyes are dry and her gaze is toward the mountain, but Abraham releases tears that have been held back since Vietnam as I take him in my arms. When the pain of a lifetime has been safely spent, I nod and they depart.*

I return to my rock to wait but find myself rudely blown from my familiar seat by an uncommon wind. I seek a sturdy tree branch to grasp as an avalanche of mighty rocks descends from the fog-drenched peak, breaking my own rock in pieces. Before the rumble ceases, there is no familiar rock in my "safe place," only rubble. I hold to my new shelter, the tree, and shake with the rocks. The tree comforts me as I had comforted Abraham.

Peace returns to the mountain but it is not long before I feel the first tremor beneath my feet. The tree shudders with me, and the rocks quake once again. The tree and I cling to each other in terror, wondering whether we will make it through the night. Neither the tree nor I have ever experienced an earthquake before. Ultimately, the ground settles and slowly we release our death grip on each other.

The thunder did not provide its usual early warning because of the other noises on the mountain tonight. No sooner have I released my hold on the tree than my friendly shelter is hit by lightning and consumed in fire. There seems to be no safe place to run to as other trees are blitzed and incinerated. The mountain burns like hell itself, and I am anxious for the small family negotiating its terrain. My impulse is to flee below to the safety of the city, but I remain and keep watch until the flames die out. There is only a charred corpse that remains of my tree.

No owl hoots. No chipmunk scurries. Even the wind has died. The silence that follows the wind, the earthquake, and fire are like the void that I imagine would follow a nuclear holocaust. Absolute silence. Then, softly, in the silence, comes a still small voice from the direction of Moriah's peak.

"Abraham?"

"Here am I, Lord!"

"Sarah, are you there, too?"

"Here I am, Lord!"

"Abraham, Sarah, I love you," the still small voice continues.

"Love us, Lord?" questions Abraham as he holds Sarah and Isaac to him.

"Sarah, whom I made to laugh because of Isaac. Abraham, the future father of many nations. Abraham! Sarah! Do you love me?"

For Viktor, who placed his visa and manuscript on the altar, the question became not whether one escapes but rather *Shema Yisrael*. For Naomi, whose passion for motherhood was on the altar, the answer was not yes or no but God's love. Before Moriah, we think we know all the answers. On Moriah we learn that we did not even know what the question was.

Epilogue:

Saying Amen

*The Spirit and the bride say, "Come." And let everyone
who hears say, "Come." And let everyone who is thirsty
come. . . . The one who testifies to these things says,
"Surely I am coming soon." Amen. Come, Lord Jesus!*
REVELATION 22:17, 20 (NRSV)

Sometimes I ask parents: "If you could rewrite the story
of your life, would you wipe out this experience without any
trace?" Although they would all omit the physical suffering of
their child, few would want to return to their former philosophy of life. A mother once confided to me that until her own
son developed leukemia, she had never thought about a single
seriously ill child. In our hospital, she opened her eyes to the
vast and varied problems that can afflict our young. Her child
had leukemia, but there were these other children with heart
failure, kidney disease, and chromosomal syndromes—organ
failure, after disease, after syndrome. She could only conclude
that either they had all been previously hidden in some closet
or her own view of the world was too narrow and protected.

Charles Hummel comments,

> The book of Job . . . gives clues to the meaning of
> suffering. But we do not really understand this

81

message—in fact, we hardly take it seriously—until we suffer. Our initial knowledge may come from the Bible, but deeper understanding comes only as we put teaching into practice.[1]

A father who lost three children in early infancy to the same miserable disease told me that he personally believed God was more than passively involved in their suffering as a family. He had belief more painful than unbelief. Yet at the emergency birth of their fourth child, realizing that once again they had lost, he postponed his own grief to organize the medical staff of a small community hospital. Thanks to this family, blood samples, placenta, and autopsy material were preserved for a research team in a distant state. They facilitated a breakthrough in the understanding of the disease that will benefit children and parents of the future, but not them directly.

This couple may have lacked answers as to *why*, but they understood *what* action their faith required of them. Parents of children with cancer unite to support each other in organizations such as "Candlelighters."[2] I hear the voices of these parents echo when I read J. B. Phillips's rendering of 2 Corinthians 4:9: "We may be knocked down but we are never knocked out!"

Eileen is another wonderful mother I know. After her son's diagnosis with leukemia, she became interested in the spiritual welfare of children and returned to graduate school for a degree in religious education. When her son relapsed and was admitted to the hospital, she used quiet moments while he slept to study. One day in his hospital room, I noticed some books written by theologians who are famous for their skeptical opinions about the miraculous stories in the Bible. I asked Eileen why she was reading those particular theologians.

"I'm taking a course entitled: 'Is the resurrection of Jesus Christ relevant today?'" I told her that I knew what those authors said about the Resurrection, but I was more interested in what she had to say. It was with great peace and joy that she looked at her seriously ill son who was laboring to breathe and answered, "I *know* that it's relevant!"

I write these words on Good Friday, one week after the death of Eileen's son. I am reminded that without the agony of the Cross, the Resurrection would have been just as irrelevant as some contemporary theologians believe it to be. It would be far easier to turn our backs on Jesus' cross and claim only his resurrection and triumph. But then we quickly lose the power of the very miracle we seek to celebrate. And we would be forgetting Jesus' admonition that we must take up our own crosses if we would follow him.

My own vision of God is more informed by these "parental theologians" I meet in my clinic than by the best and most brilliant scholars who rarely venture from the safety of their essays and books, pulpits and classrooms. David Biebel's firstborn son died in early childhood from a bizarre neurological disease, and his second son is afflicted with the same rare syndrome. In a poem entitled "Lament" this evangelical pastor asks,

Destroy! Destroy! Our little boy,
What sad, demented mind, unkind
Would dare?
GOD?[3]

When his second son was diagnosed with the same illness, he dared to articulate what he was actually feeling: "If that's the way it's going to be, then God can go to hell!"

They were honest words, but they tasted like blasphemy on his tongue. As he drove to his parents' home that night to tell them that Christopher, too, was afflicted with the illness that took Jonathan's life, he realized the ironic truth of his "blasphemous" words, and with that realization came God's comfort. On Good Friday, at the place of the skull, God *did* go to hell. As David sobbed, he sensed God's message to him: "I understand, my son. I've been there already. I've felt your pain and carried your sorrows. I know your words arose from grief beyond control and I love you still and always will."[4]

Let me return to my prayer for my young friend Tony. It was not an exercise of the head but a demand of the heart. My prayer, "Don't You care at all?" was answered in my heart as quickly as my thoughts blasted the heavens: "Yes, I do care, and it's because I care that you are there. And I am there also."

Those in the fiery furnace find One who walks with them. Those who walk through the valley of the shadow of death do not walk alone. God, the Parent who so loved the world, became a co-sufferer with all parents who share Mount Moriah's supreme test of faith, through the gift and death of his beloved Son.

Before my career is complete, there will be many more Tonys who will choke back their tears. I doubt that many of their parents will report that all of their hard theological questions found answers. Neither will I, and we continue to pose some awfully tough arguments.

At least when we challenge God, we keep a conversation going. That type of conversation is called prayer. And occasionally in the conversation, God interrupts, so to speak, and gets a word or two in edgewise. To hearts untroubled and hearts unsure, there is a window to heaven in the abiding promise that Jesus will come. *Amen. Come, Lord Jesus!*

A Child Shall Lead Them

Let Me Tell You About My Grandchildren

⚬━⋙⋘━⚬

Blessed be childhood, which brings down something of heaven into the midst of our rough earthliness.
HENRI FRÉDÉRIC AMIEL

Dear Crumb Bunny,

On the day of your bone marrow transplantation, I must tell you what a very special baby you are. And very, very blessed. Sitting by your crib, writing a letter in your Book of Hope, I imagine that you will read these words on your wedding day.

This disease that brought you to death's portal (and to my office door) comes to only one in a million babies. Most of them die. I am determined that you will be a bride.

You are special because, in a manner of speaking, you have five living grandparents. When I was born, only one of my grandparents was still alive. I will tell you how your doctor got to be your extra grandma. First, let me tell you a bedtime story, a tale of princesses and of grandmas.

A mommy asked her little girl what she wanted to be when she grew up. The child thought for a while, taking her time to

87

answer, as little girls will. "I want to be a princess," she said. "And a grandma."

"What does a princess do?" her mother inquired. Her daughter confidently replied, "A princess wears beautiful long dresses and dances all day in a wonderful castle!" Her eyes widened and she looked away, mistily and mysteriously dreaming of her future castle.

"And what does a grandmother do?" probed her mother. That took a bit more contemplation. "A grandma does the dishes and makes the beds and washes the windows . . . Maybe I'll just be a princess!¹

Let me tell you, Princess, this grandma doesn't wash windows! But grandmas have more in our job description than that little princess knew. Grandmothers are the keepers of family history and folklore. We like to link the past to the present while we rock little princesses in our ample bosoms.

To be a grandma is to be a storyteller. To be a princess is to be the story.

The headline on the early evening news was riveting: HISTORY IS BEING MADE TODAY AT YALE-NEW HAVEN HOSPITAL . We were gathered together in the Bone Marrow Transplantation Unit, savoring a moment of victory, watching a year of our collective lives unfold on television in sixty-second sound bites.

An anchorwoman titillated her viewers, warning that some of the scenes to follow would be "graphic." File footage of an operating room filled the screen with the image of a patient anesthetized upon a table, sterilely draped, poised for action. Steel needles flashed, glass syringes shimmered, dramatic tension peaked. Attention focused on the sleeping bone-marrow donor, a giver of life.

"So that's how it's done!" observed a bald man on the other side of a plastic barrier from us. "I've never seen how they actually get the bone marrow." Medical staff and family of a mortally ill baby whom I had nicknamed Crumb Bunny huddled outside a yellow line to watch the news.

It was, in fact, a patient billeted inside the protective environment of a Bone Marrow Transplant room who was speaking to us. We were his guests-at-a-safe-distance for the early evening news. A yellow line, the border of no-man's-land, separated us from this young businessman in his "life island." Were we to step over the line, his life would be in danger.

As the story unrolled, this young man himself appeared on the TV screen, the camera skillfully shooting through the protective, transparent partition. The news team had interviewed him earlier in the day and learned his own happy story. He was close to discharge time now, his brother's donated cells willingly repopulating his own empty marrow space.

A few doors away, another story was just beginning. A baby played in her crib. She, a newcomer to this alien world, had a long road ahead. We don't often have such very young children in the Bone Marrow Unit. The staff had lovingly decorated the baby's cubicle with all the care that first-time parents devote to their firstborn child's nursery. Sterile need not translate as impersonal.

But we were not the only players in this prime-time drama. Barely 200 miles away, a helicopter was meeting a British jumbo jet at Kennedy Airport, delivering our nurse Hanne and a priceless gift-harvest for the seventeen-month-old infant. Hanne hadn't bargained for a helicopter ride when she accepted the assignment to hand-carry the life-saving gift all the way from a British operating theater. We all wanted to see the blush on her cheeks when she finally landed and saw all the TV cameras and all of us.

We had waited an entire year for this day. The baby was born healthy but became sick shortly thereafter. Three years earlier, her brother died soon after birth from the same strange illness. It was not until she came to us that the correct diagnosis, a one-in-a-million genetic disease, was suspected.

For many years my research has focused on a peculiar and rare disease known as "histiocytosis." The baby had the most rare and deadly form of this disease. Until the last few years, all babies born with this form of histiocytosis, like her brother, eventually died. But now there was hope.

It was exhilarating to read the early reports in medical journals of a possible cure. Bone marrow transplantation—taking cells from a healthy brother or sister and giving it to the sick child—was a relatively new way to manage this disease. This baby had no surviving sibling, no such match. And this awful disease, held in check by chemotherapy, was starting to come back.

Sadly, we were aware of many infants who died before finding an unrelated donor. Turning from the small, intimate family circle to a vast uncaring world is an act of desperate hope. Would a stranger care enough about a stranger? Could we find a donor in time?

There was cause for celebration that evening. There was just such a caring person, thousands of miles away. A perfectly matched but unrelated bone marrow donor had been located in England, renewing hope for our baby.

Now it was time to mobilize. As we waited for the bone marrow to arrive, the staff of *Guideposts* magazine gathered in their corporate offices to pray for her. Members of the family's church organized an all-day prayer vigil. Days before, we made room in her small body for the new bone marrow with lethal doses of chemotherapy.

As she waved at me through the plastic curtain, it was hard to grasp how absolutely defenseless she was against common germs in ordinary air, clear tap water. The whir of a laminar air-flow fan was a sinister reminder of her total vulnerability.

At six o'clock we all rushed out to the hospital helipad together, waving and giggling and hugging each other like happy fools, shading our eyes from the sunset. The journalists beat us and had cameras and notebooks poised for the dramatic moment when our nurse would emerge from the chopper.

Lenses zoomed in on the delivery to Dr. Joel Rappeport, then swept to the young parents. They told of searching the world for a suitable donor for their only surviving child. Mom and Dad said they believed that this moment was an answer to prayer.

One of the media herd noticed my enthusiastic enjoyment of the moment and hoped there might be another story here to the side of the crowd. "Who are you?" she asked, "The baby's grandmother?"

My colleagues stared at her in disbelief. When she heard my name and realized who I was, she stammered an apology and mumbled her congratulations to the entire medical team.

Later that evening, my car crossed the Quinnipiac Bridge that spans my two worlds. On this twilight re-entry from high-tech hospital to hemlock-guarded hideaway, I thought about her words. Surely there must have been something in my expression that led her to conclude that I was the baby's grandmother.

What a superb compliment it was, this suspicion of grandmotherliness. And what a rare opportunity it now provides. Years ago I began talking of the offspring of my long-term surviving patients as my "grandchildren." Now that I'm getting older, even my patients' parents are young enough to be my children. If you have a few hours, dear reader, let me tell you about these grandchildren. Let me share my world with you.

Set aside your presumptions about sickness and death, children and cancer. Prepare yourself for paradox. Where you suppose death to rule, life abounds. Where you expect pathos, there may be humor in its place. Children will lead and wise adults will follow. Leave your biases at the door. And take off your shoes, for this is holy ground. But you are safe and welcome. It is only your presumptions you need to leave behind.

1

A Child Shall Lead Them

A door had opened in the universe, and through my
son, and in my face. The Glory of the Lord had burst
from a little child.

WALTER WANGERIN, JR.

Dear Crumb Bunny,

Precious, irreplaceable, vulnerable, and mortally ill you
were when we first met. I adored you at first sight, made you part
of our family. I brooded over the grim medical facts of your case and
watched my colleagues mentally hang a crêpe over your small crib.

Because of your diagnosis, my co-workers saw you as good
as dead. Statistically, they were entitled to that opinion. But I aimed
to transpose gloom into hope, hope into action. This was the genesis of your Book of Hope.

Today, your day of hope, is a time to say "thank you."
First, let me thank you for coming into my life, enriching it. But I
am not your only admirer. Taped near your crib is a card from your
donor with her blessings for you. She signed her first name, and we
have formed mental pictures of this woman we have come to love
like a sister. Your parents have organized a package of thank-you

93

notes to send her. The British bone-marrow registry will forward our thanks to her. Thus far there are more than 100 cards to send.

Babies can make adults do the most unusual things that we just won't do for each other. As long as there are babies, there will be hope.

I didn't start my medical studies intending to be a pediatrician of any sort, much less a specialist in children's cancer. Yet at 3:00 A.M. in December last year I found myself in a hospital emergency room, preparing to inflict pain on a stranger's child.

"Matt, I have to give you a shot," I prepared him as I ripped open an alcohol wipe. The medicinal sting in my nose revived a long-forgotten memory. When I was Matt's age, my own pediatrician planned to give me a simple shot of penicillin. To attempt this, he had to chase me around an examining table. The old sport wasn't up to the chase the day of my reckoning and quit after a few sweaty laps. Frustrated and irritated, he suspended further efforts to corral me. He informed my mother that my hysteria would neutralize the antibiotic even if he gave it. My adrenaline, he alleged, could undo the wonder drug's wonder. Even then I could spot a pharmacological fib.

Matt gave me a merry chase in the months that would follow his rite of passage on that bleak midwinter night. He reminded me what it is like to be a frightened child. I recall his father's love and his mother's determination. His mother will not let me give up on the chase, and I will not fib.

His mother stayed with him for all painful procedures we performed to save Matt's life. When I looked up from my instruments, I could see her practicing her tigress look. When you're a mother, you sometimes have to think with your claws.

When I finished, I saw the tears form in her eyes as she whispered "thank you."

I never considered making my baby doctor's career my own. In medical school a professor of pediatrics reinforced this disinclination. During my apprenticeship on a children's ward, I sat at a nurses' station listening to his unsolicited advice.

"Don't go into pediatrics," he advised, punctuating his professorial counsel with a paternal pat on my hand. "Women shouldn't be exposed to suffering children." He was serious. He meant to persuade.

Assurances followed. He pointed to his own daughter, a doctor. He saw himself as an authentic believer, not an arrant bigot. He saw a place for women in medicine, but not in pediatrics.

He had steered his daughter (and hoped to lead me) away from his own special field. Mysteries were safer with men, I imagined him to imagine. Rachel might weep for her children because they are no more.

Suffering and death can be deep, deep mysteries indeed. As a student, my greatest fear was that I might weep. I imagined that the faculty watched the rare women students, waiting for the waterworks to begin, and I did not want to give them ammunition for their biases.

An instructor in pharmacology was distraught when I wept over a dog we used for a laboratory experiment. The instructor said that they had never taught him in graduate school what to do about such situations. I took that to mean that he didn't know what to do about women students. Tears and chaos that had erupted in his lab.

I caught his facial expression and never wept again. I thought of that day as I listened to my newest instructor. Was this pediatrician a prophet, anticipating the dark night of the soul ahead for me? Or was he simply a kinder and gentler sexist?

The scene at the nurses' station so long ago was one of those magic moments of mentoring, how young doctors learn the art of medicine. We learn by the example of others, what they choose to share. Thirty years later, at a different nurses' station in another hospital, I am the baby doctor, the professor, the mentor. I face a suffering boy who must suffer more before daylight comes. A young medical student sits near me, observing my every move.

My earnest dissuader in medical school was the first but not my only instructor in the health care of children. In that mammoth city hospital, young pediatricians-in-training tried to persuade me to join their happy ranks. The pediatric residents were happy zealots, looking for new comrades.

Pediatrics was one of the few departments in that teaching hospital without a jail ward. In that sprawling haven for the suffering poor, there never were enough beds for all those in need. Prison bars may have been missing from the outer perimeters of the pediatric wards, but the lives of many of the little ones were similarly governed by circumstances over which they had no control.

Trapped by poverty, the parents seemed as powerless as their babes. In this department where you learned how to change diapers before you learned how to change medication orders, I met senior doctors who were convinced that they could make a difference in a sad, sad world. And the most outrageous Don Quixote of them all was in charge.

The chief pediatrician had high expectations of us all. He assumed that we knew the scientific issues. He was more interested to hear what we had learned as human beings. He wasn't content to let invisible bars confine him and the babes in his charge. Once he had even taken on City Hall on behalf of youngsters whose bones and brains were filled with an urban poison. Lead poisoning could be today's death or tomorrow's learning disability, but this doctor simply would not let the children go home to die by either route.

As medical students, we could recite all the biochemical esoterica, the enzymatic blocks by which the damage is done. But if we had no comprehension of the social implications of the illness—of how lead actually got into the systems of these children—we had failed in his view.

The pediatric bed-census validated his claims. Our wards were always full of these children, long after they were well enough for discharge. Tenement housing, the source of their ailments, had low priority with the bureaucrats. One month before I started pediatrics, I completed an assignment in community health, visiting a family who lived in this sort of subsidized squalor. The building was so dangerous that we sometimes borrowed a friend's German shepherd to make our house calls. Today, you would need an armed police escort.

I have seen firsthand the chips of old lead-based paint that peel off the walls and find their way into hungry mouths, growing brains. No one listened to the impoverished tenants when they complained. They were welfare clients, after all. Their caseworkers reminded them of how fortunate they were to even have a roof over their heads.

A "hot line" linked Dr. Lanman's office to the Health Department laboratory where they tested blood lead levels. He refused to discharge a child from our hospital until the housing was safe. Since the city could not afford for our acute beds to be filled with chronic cases, an inspector was promptly dispatched to the home to facilitate repairs. This good doctor used his power to assist the powerless and won.

My hero was a dashing silver fox in long, white cotton twill. We murmured to each other as he strode down the hall, recounting tales of all the windmills he had successfully slain. I was the chief murmurer.

❦

On the pediatric wards I felt free to be myself. My infatuation with a baby hospitalized for heart problems was no great secret. Her mother was so afraid that Milagros would die that she never visited her child. When the nurses called me about her medical care, they would refer to me as her "mother."

My own income was below poverty level that year, but I bought a secondhand sewing machine and made elegant lace-trimmed nightgowns for my lovely new Hispanic "daughter." I was always partial to lace, and so was Milly. She was very proud and pranced in her crib, fussing with the lace.

I always assumed that my extra-curricular stitches were my secret, known only to the nurses. My assumption proved flawed when the senior doctors joined us one day for rounds. As we came to Milly's crib, I stood to the rear of the group lest the baby and the nurses betray me.

The chief unbuttoned the lace ribbon at her neckline to listen to her heart. Then he turned to find me. "Dr. Komp, I recognize your suturing when I see it. I assume that you will be carrying this baby along with us for the rest of our rounds. The next time, just get her before we start. Milly shouldn't have to wait so long for her 'mother' to collect her."

This regal gentleman did not pat hands. If he was a father figure, he was the sort who blessed and released. He blessed me by his example and released me to chart my own way. Yet I still had no serious thoughts about pediatrics for my own career.

❦

Never did I hear a word of direct advice from my next teacher, the person whose opinion meant the most to me. For four happy weeks I worked with an eminent physician who had escaped from Cuba to start his professional life over in America.

Although trained as an internist, Ramon Torres became a heart specialist for children and found himself most at home with youngsters and their advocates. To complete his American credentials, he had to step away from a senior faculty position for a year and become a resident. When I was a student, he was my supervising pediatric resident. I followed him everywhere, and he simply taught me everything that he knew about children.

Would I choose internal medicine or pediatrics? I agonized over the necessary choice until the deadline for internship applications came due. The younger residents tried to coax; Torres never said a word.

I cannot remember the exact sequence of thoughts that led to the most important career decision I've ever made. It seemed as if the heavens had opened and a big sign with the word PEDIATRICS emblazoned upon it was lowered for my viewing. I ran to Dr. Torres' office with the revelation.

"Diane, Diane!" he laughed, shaking his head. "You were the only one who didn't know you were going into pediatrics." That day I completed my applications for a pediatric residency, a decision I've never regretted.

Now, at 3:00 A.M., I am in another hospital with a different pediatric resident at my side. He is weary from long hours, worried about Matt, and very alarmed at the diagnosis I suspect. The yellow cast to the child's skin, the balloon-tight belly, his pain-haunted eyes—they all spell malignancy. Not school phobia as the first doctor suspected, nor hepatitis as the second one had hoped.

This young resident chose pediatrics because he supposed that children only get quick-fix illnesses, if they get sick at all. Sneeze one day, play the next. Cancer is an obscenity that should happen to no one, much less a child. Neither should a stranger inflict more pain on a little stranger. Nor should parents need to scrutinize a doctor's eyes in search of truth and hope. I know his thoughts (they once were mine).

Our job together, learner and mentor, is to fight for Matt's life. In striving together all night this night, hopefully, I will pass on something worth learning. And I will not pat his hand.

My career "revelation" solved one dilemma, but it left another in its place. The mystery of suffering continued to loom, unresolved, threatening. Because of my own choice, no one could protect me from little ones who suffer. But I still demanded an answer about their suffering. Both science and religion had led me to believe that questions had answers. My quest led past the children and their parents—to God. And there the buck stopped . . . with God.

Beholding the mystery, my faith began to flounder. A boy with hemophilia injured himself every Christmas to come to our hospital. Our "home" was happier than his. Leukemia filled a little girl's brain, leaving her with hallucinations about horrible bugs crawling on her skin. We gave her a tranquilizer. The imaginary bugs remained, but she no longer cared. Where was the hope for these children?

Surely, lambs and lions could not lie together, as some silly prophet had once declared! From my vantage point, God seemed to be flogging the lambs instead of the lions. How could a rational person believe in such a deity? How shall I find my own way in this jungle, much less lead little lambs to safety?

What lay ahead in the jungle for me was to learn that it was not I who would lead the children home. *It would be the children who would lead me instead.*

2

Let My Heart Be Broken

The heart must break or become as bronze.

CHAMFORT

Dear Crumb Bunny,

I asked all your doctors and nurses to write notes in your Book of Hope for you to read when you grow up. To envision you grown up—Crumb Bunny in a bridal gown rather than a burial shroud—takes a leap of faith. In recent years, faith has not been a notable component of medical tradition.

As they struggled to find the words for your Book of Hope, I watched the attitude on the ward miraculously start to change. I saw a subtle, even a hopeful progression in the notes they entered in your medical chart as well. Doctors and nurses joined us in the sweet conspiracy, the daring hope, the outrageous consideration that you might survive. They did not want their hearts to be broken.

When I was little, they used to say about a particularly sweet girl-child that when she grew up she would break men's hearts. You, little flirt, have those kinds of looks. But of you they say, "If she doesn't grow up, it will break my heart."

There are many adults I know who try to shield themselves from such heartbreak. Your mother, dear child, is not one of them. For a child, her own or someone else's, she will always take a risk.

There's a sweetness to your mom that I hope you have inherited. As sick as you are and as sad as your own family's story has been, she has always cared about all the children who come to our clinic. Your mother's attitude reminds me of a saying I heard many years ago: "Let my heart be broken with the things that break the heart of God."

Perhaps my first pediatric teacher was right. To be exposed to suffering children is a dangerous proposition. As children died, my faith seemed to perish as well. To handle the pain, I took the advice of a professor of internal medicine.

He was doing his best to counsel young students as he rounded with us on our patients. He advised us not to heed the pain that our feelings bring when we listen to our patients. We should simply do our work and concentrate on that. Hard work is a good tonic for untamed and uneasy feelings. There was plenty of work, ample opportunity to concentrate away from the untidy arena of emotion.

Yet there's a critical distinction between suspending feelings for the moment and denying that they ever mattered. This professor never tried to make such a distinction, but I believe he shared as best he knew. Feelings are the purview of social workers, not doctors, he thought.

Empathy, what most patients long for from their doctors, is defined as "the identification with, and understanding of another's situation, *feelings*, and motives."[1] For me, the denial of full-bodied empathy to my patients was a personal loss as well. It spelled the difference between spiritual life and death.

True empathy resonates with life's most profound questions. It is only when we share the feelings of another that we understand the importance of hope. *Without hope, we cannot live. Without hope, we are already dead.* Of course, we could choose work that keeps us away from dying patients altogether. Where is it written, thou shalt be a masochist?

I learned to work unflogged by untidy feelings. But every time I considered taking a "safe" course, to avoid the suffering of children, the path led away from the most joyous parts of medicine as well. There were mysteries within the mystery.

There was a particular boy with leukemia I met when I was an intern, who seemed destined to die. *If he must die*, I thought, *let it be peaceful.* An oncologist came along with a drug so new that it was still considered investigational. Vincristine was unlikely to cure his disease, but it was certain to make his hair fall out. I wondered about this peculiar breed of pediatricians who gave "poisons" to mere babes. We students and residents gossiped about these ghouls behind their backs, yet they seemed to be the only members of the faculty that we saw after midnight. Their patients and the parents received them as members of the family, even seemed to love them. Their words and their protocols brought hope, it seemed. *There must be something about their job*, I thought, *that we fledgling baby-docs do not yet understand.*

It was this speciality that attracted me most, even though it threatened the most exposure to suffering children. Remember, this was a quarter century ago, when few children with cancer survived these treatments. It defies logic why I made the choice.

I entered the speciality with the intention to pursue laboratory-based work, safe from baldness and tears. I also reasoned that this would be the likeliest place to find a solution to the puzzle of disease. This was the sort of hope a scientist could understand. In my childhood, science had saved us from polio. Now science could address the next important plague of children: cancer.

But science failed regularly. I risked drowning in a sea of malignant ifs. If I were smarter. If I had read just one more article. If I had stayed up a few more hours. Rather than drown, I swam back to the safety of the lab. When I did work with the kids, I did my best, secure in the knowledge that I could keep my safe distance. Someone else was ultimately responsible.

As a junior faculty member, I was able to maintain this distance until an unexpected turn of events. The colleague who did most of the clinical work in our department left for another medical school. But his patients stayed behind.

At first I made plans to recruit another doctor to take care of the clinical work. To my amazement, I found that the closer I got to children with cancer, the easier the job was. Instead of sapping my energy, these kids were life-giving. The malignant ifs were transmuted into peace of mind. Gladly, the job close to the children became mine.

Instead of expecting a miracle worker, the children with cancer and their parents seemed satisfied with a fellow sojourner. If I did my best, that sufficed. What was important to them was that we were there together. One young mother and her firstborn son made a profound impression on me. So vivid is my memory of her that I used her for the prototype for Sarah in *A Window to Heaven*.

It was this young family who motivated me to support home care for dying children long before we in America heard about hospice. It was children like her own who showed me a window to heaven, full of hope, dreams, visions, and faith.

From this young mother I learned that there are wiser teachers than the professors. You can recognize them by the diaper bags they carry. Near the time of her son's death, she spoke of another young doctor who suffered because of her own sense of inadequacy. "I wanted to tell her that she would be okay—that there would be another patient for her to care for. But of course, at the time I couldn't find the words to say." *My professors were not half as wise as she.*

Today more than half of young people diagnosed with cancer will survive without any evidence of disease recurrence. The news is especially good for children with some forms of leukemia where the expectations are that 80 percent of them will live to tell the story about their victories. There is even better news about infants with a common form of malignant tumor when limited to the kidney. For them, the cure rate approaches 100 percent. Every year the report gets better. Even for Matt.

Matt went directly from Emergency to our Intensive Care Unit. My worst fear was realized when the biopsy came back as Burkitt's lymphoma. This malignancy grows so fast that some of these children die in the first few days. The first early days were not very pleasant, but Matt's parents were there at his side. That made all the unpleasantries doable.

It takes many different doctors and a team of nurses to pull such a child through. When the chemo started to work, both Matt's health and smile returned. He has a wonderful, nine-year-old boy's smile, auguring mischief as well as remission. Six months later, his treatment is complete. No Burkitt's cells can be found.

Matt celebrates his latest good report by joining a panel of adult cancer survivors, telling participants in an international congress that they can ask him any questions they desire. There's no question too painful if he can help someone else. He is happy to be there; his parents beam with pride. On my twenty-fifth anniversary as a pediatric oncologist, I am proud as well.

The good news does not stop with the improvements in treatment. Supported by the company of the children, I started to ask questions again of God. I heard no voice from heaven, but I did hear the voice of the children. It was through their voices that I understood what Jesus meant when he said, "And remember, I am with you always, to the end of the age" (Matt. 28:20). *These are words full of hope.*

I have never regretted the choice of oncology for a career. It's been my privilege to participate in three of the fastest-moving decades in cancer treatment and make my own small contributions to the progress. It is not professional success that keeps me in the field. It is the children.

Tonight I think back on the pain that I tried to avoid by distancing myself from these children and realize how much greater the pain of avoidance is than that of their embrace. I hear the echo of my own once-breaking heart in a voice on my telephone answering-machine.

It was hard to hear the entire message because of the choked-back tears that punctuated his words. My caller was a middle-aged man who identified himself as a pastor in the Midwest. He was distraught. A child in his congregation had an aggressive tumor, and nothing in seminary or three decades of parish ministry had prepared him for this painful experience. He had never dealt with a child with cancer before.

As we spoke, he stammered with emotion but managed to tell me about the child's family. Their community doctor had sent them to a major pediatric cancer center. The staff of the big center were marvelous and supportive, he said. The parents were doing fine. He referred to them as "bearers of the holy." But the pastor's heart was breaking. A member of his church was suffering, and he felt impotent. He seemed to be suffering more than the sufferer.

A pastor weeps. Yet parents rise up with wings as eagles. Young doctors with other options count themselves privileged to cast their lot with these children. And middle-aged physicians like me can find our way back to faith when we listen to such children.

Therein is the paradox: *The closer you come to these children, the less the pain. If you risk your heart being broken, you just may find it healed.*

3

Isaac's Return
from Mount Moriah

⟨≈❦≈⟩

*This strange tale is about fear and faith, fear and defi-
ance, fear and laughter. Terrifying in content, it has
become a source of consolation to those who, in
retelling it, make it part of their own experience.*

ELIE WIESEL

Dear Crumb Bunny,

Unlike a medical chart, your Book of Hope is beautiful
enough for a bride. This floral-fabric journal is your hospital guest-
book for visitors. The book was my idea, but it was your mother's
notion to bring hope into its title. My billets-doux are a different
type of medical progress note.

Your story, little one, reminds me of a biblical one, of
Abraham and Isaac on the path up to Mount Moriah. As the story
goes, God asked a man of faith to sacrifice his only living son that
he loved. St. Paul said that Abraham hoped against hope that Isaac
would survive.

You may have noticed that your parents are people of faith. But would they take you and risk your life if they did not trust God? For most parents, the analogy of Mount Moriah is incomplete. Few parents I meet as a doctor get to exercise free choice. Most just find themselves there on the mountain, forced to decide under pressure. Your own Abraham and Sarah know the metaphor in full.

As long as you were sick, the decision to accept the chemotherapy was an easy one. There was no other choice for sane parents. They made a date to deliver you up, signed consent for lethal doses of even more powerful drugs to be administered to wipe out your own bone marrow. This is strong stuff for doctors, let alone parents.

The medications to destroy your own bone marrow began days before Nurse Hanne winged her way over to London. What if the donor had second thoughts and backed out? What if Hanne tripped and dropped the container with the marrow?

Mommy and Daddy hope against hope. They are at peace with God's loving care for you.

In *A Window to Heaven* I drew on the story of Mount Moriah to describe the plight of parents in such a situation. The majority of the children I wrote about in that book did not return from the Mount. This book has a different emphasis, so my metaphoric Isaac shall return.

A few small rocks are the first to break the silence, and then an unmodulated voice of a young lad is heard as he races down the hillside. Sarah's voice echoes as she calls after him, "Isaac! Don't run so fast. You haven't even walked for a month. Isaac! Where are you?"

His face is flushed with excitement as he races up to me. "Dr. Di, did you see what happened on the mountain? Awesome!

Hey, I'm hungry. I could eat a whole cow. You got any peanut butter crackers? Awesome!"

Sarah and Abraham reach the foot of the mountain, nod to me briefly, and then head for home. There are no words that need to be said. Their Isaac is safe.

Snug in his bed, surrounded by a legion of stuffed animals, Isaac snores softly. Sarah sits on the edge of the bed running her fingers through his curly hair. It had been straight before the treatment, but now there are these handsome curls.

The first stage is what we call the "chemo cut." In the summer, the chemo cut bleaches out on the tips. It's hard to overcome the temptation to run your fingers through the thick pelt that eventually replaces the bald pate.

Little boys roll their eyes when mothers and doctors give in to the tactile temptation. In this sense we love being weak. As the child sleeps soundly, Sarah's resolve that never was dissolves. Her fingers plow rows through the dense rich crown. They are a symbol of hope.

Abraham joins her and they watch Isaac sigh. In his sleep, he clutches the teddy bear he got after his last bone marrow transplant. One for every marrow, another for each spinal, Isaac sleeps in a zoological garden. When he goes off to college, Sarah will take teddy and the others to her own room before her son discards them in a fit of pubertal machismo.

In the marital bed, Abraham and Sarah embrace each other tightly to shut out all that is not them and theirs and allow their eyes to overflow. Tears of relief, streams of repressed anger, rivers of joy flow that they have returned from Moriah with their family intact. Then their embrace broadens and with it their prayers for other families. Mostly they pray for Isaac, that he will always know how special he is to God. Then they sleep.

Sarah and Abraham will never forget where they have been, nor what has happened. Chances are that Isaac's memory will fade as he grows up.

Woody, a lively child, was just short of his third birthday when he developed leukemia and came into my care. Without coaching, he tuned out the pain from bone marrows and spinal taps. I gloved, and he snored. It was that simple. He never felt a thing.

When he was a mature man of five, he forgot all that and couldn't understand what we were talking about when we tried to remind him. Our social worker thought that nursery rhymes might be a suitable trick to help him regain what he had lost. An indignant preschooler listened suspiciously, then sputtered out, "I don't want no rock. I want Mozart!" For the next two years, I did his bone marrows to *Eine kleine Nachtmusik*. Again, he never felt a thing.

Time passed and he became an old gent of twelve. When I told him that he needed a bone marrow, he howled and haggled. He shook his head at me once more, "You keep telling me about putting myself to sleep and doing bone marrows to Mozart. I don't remember that at all." His parents and I will always remember and wish he did, too.

In the land that gave us Sigmund Freud, I shared this story with pediatricians. The members of the Austrian Pediatric Society were less impressed with the point I intended to make about pain control than the musical message. In America there dwells one small child who prefers Mozart to rock!

I've known Woody for most of his life. He is proud that he is no longer a little boy. I've seen him grow into new skills but I've also seen him outgrow some of his earliest abilities. Woody has reached an age when he needs to be retaught some things that he once seemed to know intuitively. I wonder what or Whom he knew that helped him so much when he was so young.

I heard a story recently about a three-year-old who wanted to spend time with his new baby brother. "I want to be alone with the baby," he insisted. We can only wonder what concerns of sibling rivalry raced through his parents' minds as they listened to this modest but pregnant request.

The child was so earnest that they allowed him to remain alone in the room with the sleeping baby. With a sense of awe, he gently touched the baby and then begged quietly, "You've got to tell me about God. I'm beginning to forget already."

Parents or religious instructors are not children's true teachers. This holy imagination, a sense of spiritual origins, is intuitive in the very young. It is as if a veil descends thereafter, leaving the pilgrim in search of ways to reconnect. We older pilgrims must seek others who know the Story to tell us, too, if we would learn to hope.

Sometimes, as death approaches, the veil seems to lift in part, giving hints of that beyond, visions of angels, of Jesus, of heaven. Most of us are pilgrims in between, living with a sense of déjà vu, groping our way back to God.

❧

In her book, *Chasing the Dragon*, Jackie Pullinger tells a remarkable story about a four-year-old Chinese boy who was pronounced dead after a drowning accident.[1]

Later, he woke and told his mother of a man who had held out his hand and pulled him out of the water. His mother asked him if he knew the man's name, assuming that it was the headmaster of the school where the accident had occurred. "Don't you know?" replied the boy. "It's Jesus."

This family had fled from mainland China to Taiwan and never had contact with Christians. His mother, who had never before heard the name of Jesus, became a Christian as a result of this child's experience. What I find most remarkable is the further history of the little boy.

Although his mother became a Christian, the boy himself went on to become a drug dealer. It was in a Hong Kong prison that Miss Pullinger met him. Despite his early "inspiring" experience, he himself had to reach rock bottom as an adult before his own life was changed spiritually.

Children who survive near-fatal illnesses are no more guaranteed than the rest of us to retain God-consciousness. Isaac returns from Moriah a healthier lad, but he, too, must choose to become faithful. Isaac must become a consenting adult to the life of faith himself for the covenant to be carried forward.

4

Beating the Odds

My doctor's favorite plant is the hedge.
FROM *A CHILD WITH CANCER*,
QUOTED BY ERMA BOMBECK

Dear Crumb Bunny,

You peek through the layers of plastic that separate us until you can find me. Then you smile and give one of your backward waves, admiring your own fingers, the way you always wave. There must be an interesting secret engraved on the palm of your hand that you don't yet choose to share. Will you ever wave the way that other babies do?

I am not a betting person, and Sweetie, let me tell you something else. Jimmy, the Greek and most doctors won't be betting on you this month. You are what they call a "long shot."

Hope doesn't like to be estimated. It prefers to be non-quantitatively enjoyed. The TV journalists pressed Dr. Joel into making an on-camera guess at your odds. Reluctantly, he said "50/50." We have a choice in how we interpret these odds. We can either see your glass as half empty or half full.

A year ago your chances were closer to zero, but here you are. Now you know why I hedge. I don't like statistics. You are a princess, not a race horse. When Joel looks at you, he gives you a 100 percent look. He seems to be by you 100 percent of his time these days.

What do you want to be when you grow up besides a princess and a grandma? I always think about your surviving, entitled to your dreams. Despite the deadly nature of your illness, I have always seen you as a living person. You are someone just like me; we are not different. One day you shall die; one day I shall die. Even there, we do not differ.

So, my love, what do you want to be when you grow up? Most of my patients imagine becoming doctors, play with stethoscopes as toys, and beg us for the biggest syringes we can find. They make the best squirt guns. Their dolls all have Hickman catheters under their dresses or IVs taped on their arms. You watch us and turn our medical mysteries into your play.

I think you children will do a better job than most of us when you take our place. You certainly seem to have the heart for people. What do you carry away from us about life and death? What can you children offer your doctors to heal our own fear of death?

When I was in medical school, few children with cancer survived, and "cure" was not a word we used in the discussion of leukemia. I learned early not to play the numbers game.

As a resident, I dreaded the admission of a child with cancer to my ward and worried over what to say. Even as a young faculty member, I avoided statistics in discussing prognosis. Until recently, Crumb Bunny's disease was 100 percent fatal, and in many hospitals it still is.

Today in my office I have the privilege to see many young people who had cancer but are now what we call "long-term survivors." They have completed their treatment and are going on with their lives. When many of them first were ill, the percentages didn't promise much. But here they are today, 100 percent here. I offer them annual appointments until they want to "fire" me for an internist. Most of them stay on unless they move out of the area.

Recently, there was close to a convention of long-term survivors at my clinic. I had a bumper-crop of college freshmen this year, the sort who passionately celebrate life. These kids easily mix with the younger new ones, playing the big brother or sister. *They are a living memorial to the power of hope.*

The chemo room that they once dreaded no longer holds power over them—they are not the ones hooked up to the tubing. But it was in just such a room that they became survivors. If they can help someone else who is just starting in, they will. For the sake of another, their old fear is canceled and they cross the threshold that once brought a bilious taste to their mouths.

When I left my previous academic post to come to Yale, I entitled my last "grand rounds" there, "Pediatric Cancer: Beating the Odds." Three of my long-term survivors participated in that teaching conference. By odds, none of them should be alive. There was something particularly mean about each of their tumors that said at the outset that the odds were against them. All of these kids had outlived cancer and were off therapy for several years at the time they shared the podium with me.

A decade later I was reminded of that particular grand rounds by a telephone call on my birthday. Although I hadn't seen him for ten years, his voice was unmistakable. How can you forget the voice of the first leukemia patient you were able to tell that he was cured? Freddie was also the first of my long-term survivors to become a parent and supply me with "grand-children" to brag about.

Freddie started with leukemia as a teenager. He is now forty years old and a coal miner. In the town where he lived, only the mines provided health benefits for someone with a history of malignancy. Freddie was realistic and in love. He didn't want to jeopardize his young family.

When Freddie was first sick, his father tried to withhold the truth from him and even denied to him that he had leukemia. The son rebelled by not taking all his prescribed med-ications. When he confided this to me years later, he told me that he knew that his father meant well. But his dad had not handled the situation in a way that was in his best interests.

I thought that this was an important message, one worth sharing with other parents who face the same situation that his father faced. I arranged to videotape an interview with Freddie. As things worked out, this did not take place until after the death of his father and the birth of his first child. I have never been able to use the video for its intended purpose.

On-camera I heard that parents always know what is best for their children; parents are always right. Teenagers, on the other hand, don't know what they're talking about; they should be obedient and grateful. Now that Freddie's own children are teenagers, I wonder what he was experiencing that day of my birthday that lead him to reach out by telephone to someone who was important to him when he was the age of his children?

His children, my first "grandchildren," are already teenagers and there have been dozens more born since then to other patients. More than one is named Diane. I pulled out the details of those old grand rounds on my birthday, enjoying the excuse to reminisce.

Harold was only three years old when he had Hodgkin's disease. Thereafter, it recurred many times despite

117

treatment. His parents agreed to try a brand-new medication as part of a research trial. This drug had much the same status that vincristine had when I was an intern—unproven, not all side effects yet known. There was nothing else we could offer. This time I was the "ghoul," and new interns wondered if I had lost all common sense.

Harold not only achieved permanent remission, he has been disease-free now for twenty years. The medication he received, a new drug from Italy called adriamycin, proved to be one of the most important drugs in the history of chemotherapy. We had no way to know that then. We could only hope. Harold's mother called me a few years ago, simply to say, "I love you."

John was three when he developed lung metastases from a kidney tumor. He was already receiving the best chemotherapy we knew. I find it ironic as I reread the opening section of my grand rounds:

I want you to picture yourself as a parent. Your beautiful three-year-old daughter has not been her usual self. She appears tired and sallow to you, so you take her to your physician. . . . After an anxious wait, the verdict comes in from the laboratory. Your physician explains to you that this disease from which she suffers has no cure—but there are medications available to which 90–100 percent of similarly afflicted children respond. Once the disease remits, however, it will be necessary to continue medication or the disease will relapse.

The medication is not without side effects. The chances are now better than ever, you are told, that your daughter will live to adulthood. If she becomes pregnant, however, her pregnancies will be considered high risk; fetal wastage is a strong possibility, and birth defects have been reported in a significant number of offspring of mothers who have been similarly treated.

    You, as a parent, ask what will happen if no treatment is given. Spontaneous remissions are rare, you are told, and without treatment, your daughter most certainly will die. What is your choice? How would you weigh the preview of the quality of your child's life? Why not allow her to slip away now rather than risk toxic treatment of an "incurable" disease with potential for death at a later point?

    The radiologist who read John's chest film glared at me as he looked at the white shadow on a black background. There was no doubt that it was a tumor. He assumed that I would send him home to die and was shocked to hear my plans.

    "What do you mean, you're going to give more chemotherapy and radiotherapy? He's only three years old and he has no hope." John completed treatment twenty years ago. He plans to apply to medical school, and his mother threatens to send him to live with me to cut down on expenses.

    The rest of the introduction to that grand rounds extends the irony by inviting the audience to imagine how they would choose:

    Would your choice (for or against treatment) be influenced by the fact that the hypothetical child I described has not cancer but diabetes? We Americans have been taught to fear cancer, and the first battle in the war against cancer is against our own attitudes.

    The irony is that although John was cured of cancer, he later became a diabetic. He finds more hassles in life from insulin than he ever did from our treatment, more rigidity in lifestyle and no end of the new "chemotherapy" in sight.

I lecture about long-term survivors to each new group of medical students that comes through pediatrics at Yale. I can see from their faces that most of them prefer memorizing the odds that someone will make it than tasting the sweetness of individual victories. "That's very nice, but how representative is that case?"

Not all of them feel that way, though. I watch their faces and can now pick out from their ranks a special type of young person who is being seen in increasing numbers in medical classrooms. Although their classmates cannot tell who they are, I can spot a long-term survivor of childhood cancer five minutes into that lecture.

A Yale undergraduate sat in my office with his eyes downcast. A relative called me to ask if I could speak to Jay. After the boy finished treatment, his parents never again spoke of the experience. Jay grew up sensing that there was a family secret, that he must always bear the mark of a survivor in silence. In college he took a course on Holocaust Literature taught by Elie Wiesel and asks me, "Why did that feel so relevant?"

There were times that Jay tried to ask, but his parents always changed the subject. "Why am I flunking out of college," he asks me without pausing for a response. "God only knows that I'm smart enough and I want to be a doctor more than anything in the world. But everytime I get in a biology class, my pulse races and my hands become clammy."

For an agonizing hour he poured out his young-ancient soul. Then he rose from the chair with tears pouring down his face. "You're the best doctor I've ever met," he exclaimed. "No one has ever helped me as much as you have. How can I thank you?" I had never gotten to say a word to Jay. I had only listened.

Jay spoke of "being saved for a purpose" and having "passed from death to life." He left my office without looking back. I didn't hear from him for another year. Then, he reappeared on my doorstep without tears and looked me straight in the eyes. "When I left here, I knew what I had to do. I determined that I wouldn't come back until it was accomplished. I went back to the hospital where I was treated and asked them why they had never anticipated my problems and counseled me. *Why didn't they tell me that I had reason to hope?* But I have to give them credit for their answer."

His doctors said that they had learned from their mistakes and invited him to join them for the summer to interview other survivors. "Be a part of the solution, Jay."

He made his choice. Today Jay is an oncologist himself and speaks to others with cancer about being saved for a purpose.

5

Children Who Chisel

~※~

> How they cut loose together, David and Yahweh,
> whirling around before the ark in such a passion that
> they caught fire from each other and blazed up in a sin-
> gle flame of such magnificence.
>
> FREDERICK BUECHNER

Dear Crumb Bunny,

I love to watch you playing in your crib when I come to visit. You casually look up at me from your work, remind me that you know that I know that your work matters as much as mine.

I take my breaks, and you do, too. You want to watch boys and girls singing and dancing, so you keep standing and pointing to the TV. For you to "watch" means to take control, climb in front of the video, run it even with your IV hooked up.

Dad lifted you onto the bedside table so you could be in charge. What you can't accomplish for yourself, you assigned to your willing slaves. Neither my work nor Dad's work is more important than these moments of serfdom for you.

You are like little David standing before mighty Goliath. I don't think it even enters your mind that anything could keep you from reaching your goal.

For the past year your parents have kept their eyes on a single goal. There were many potential obstacles in their way, but they never paid them serious attention; they only concentrated on this bone-marrow transplantation. And they slew a gaggle of giants along the way.

On your honeymoon, perhaps, you could travel to Florence and see the great statue of David created by Michelangelo. You giant-slayers should get to know each other.

At his request, I visited an adult patient in our hospital, a man who was bedridden by widespread cancer. Before his chemotherapy was started, he had suffered incredible pain that not even morphine could abate.

Thanks to effective treatment, the pain was now under control, but he found the thought of a lifetime of such drugs overwhelming. He didn't see how he could face it. He had lost all hope.

In a moment of despair, he cried out, "I wish I could just end it all with a lethal injection!" A psychiatrist was summoned, a two-page typewritten note appeared in the chart testifying to his visit. Oddly (but not so oddly), he never asked this depressed young man what he believed about death and suicide.

The patient asked to see me because he wanted to know how my children manage. This question made me focus on the children, consider things I have come to take for granted. "Do you believe that the chemotherapy is helping you?" I asked.

"Oh yes!" he replied. "The first day you came to visit me I couldn't even think straight. It was the chemo that took away the pain. I'm not even on morphine now."

"It's not necessary to make a commitment to take chemotherapy for the rest of your life. Start by getting rid of that obstacle. What happens to you for the rest of your life is your choice. Do you think you could handle one cycle?" A cycle of chemotherapy was five days of treatment followed by a three-week rest period.

He looked somewhat relieved but still less than convinced. An intravenous line dripped as we spoke. "Let's break it down further," I proposed. "Can you deal with chemo today?" He nodded vigorously, remembering that his baby daughter would soon come through the door. His day revolved around her visits.

"That is how my patients think of things, in terms of today. One day at a time. Break it down into blocks of time that you know that you can deal with instead of taking on the whole thing now. *Break it down to the hope that you have.*"

"I can do that!" he exclaimed. "One day at a time. Yes, I can do that." That week, he was able to make his choice and remained at peace with it, day by day, for the rest of his life.

There is a story told about the great sculptor Michelangelo. He was once asked how he took a big hunk of marble and turned it into his masterpiece David. His answer, as I recall, was something like this: "In the marble I saw David, and I chiseled away everything that wasn't David." The artist didn't see the obstacles; he only saw his goal. The obstacles fell away like just so much rubble as he kept his eyes on David.

Occasionally I take a break and sit in the chemo room to see how the children are chiseling away. Often I see a masterpiece come into view. They have such a different view of the world from adults, worthy of our attention and consideration. I think about the tools they use and wonder what we as adults can adopt and adapt.

It is not that their obstacles are markedly different from our own. They share our pain and fears, but they do not bear them alone. They tend and feed their important relationships. Children sustain life-giving connections by revealing who they are. No smoke screens here, persona rather than person on display. What you see is what you get. Theologian Paul Minear captures it this way:

> For, to a child, it is more important to be known than to know. The ground of his confidence depends less upon how much he knows about his family than upon the inner awareness that he is known by his family. The psalmist's testimony, "O Lord, thou hast searched me, and known me" (Ps. 139:1), articulates such awareness, an awareness which rises to a climax in the Christian consciousness of being "foreknown," and in the expectation, "Then shall I know fully even as also I was fully known." (1 Cor. 13:12)[1]

These little ones love with an unconditional *agape* love. I wish that physicians who care for adults had equal access to the sort of love that the children bring. They give me the room I need to be the peculiar human being I am. Who I am need not be an obstacle to them.

Relationships are so important to children that they do their best to repair any damage quickly. Their tears quickly point to a relationship at risk. I've had to do many painful things to children over the years, but I've never left a treatment room feeling that the pain was carried away as a grievance. The child's outward expression of pain assists me, poor wretched bumbling adult that I am. I am sure to set things right before the visit ends.

Far more important than the children's opinion of me is their love for their families. Children who die do so without the need for deathbed reconciliations. It is as if their slates are clean. They remind me of the need on a daily basis to set my own accounts straight. They remind me both to ask for and offer forgiveness if I would become a child for the sake of the kingdom of heaven.

Their masterpieces (and the children themselves) are often liberated as Michelangelo's was, by creative imagination. They engage outward talents to tell an inner story. Sometimes I see them retell the story of their cancer in ways that give them power over the marble-like obstacles in their lives.

Rusty symbolizes his cancer as Mount Krebs. He sketches in a multinational counterstrike force against which the tumor cannot hope to prevail. The Red Baron and Snoopy are there, symbolizing the red color of adriamycin and the nurse who massages his shoulders when he is in the hospital. This time Snoopy and the Baron get to work together, partners on Rusty's Dream Team. Group Leader Rusty himself pilots a Sopwith Camel.

Each part of his treatment, every important human and even his dog, are all symbolized in this vintage montage. Mount Krebs shall surely fall! He proudly shows me his work, and I note the life-giving light in which he bathes his strike force. There is no darkness here.

Although our powers of creative imagination diminish with age, not even adults are a total loss. If you doubt your abilities, find your own Rusty. Or Ronnie. They will guide your feeble hand.

Ronnie came to us from another hospital in need of further testing, including a bone marrow aspirate. A young colleague learned from the family that their Christian faith was very important to them. He wondered if I could use that to help Ronnie help himself.

I decided to tap Ronnie's creative imagination and suggested that he imagine Jesus in the room helping him. "Think about Jesus. Invite him into the room. When we do something to you, I want you to squeeze Jesus tightly. I also want you to imagine that Jesus is hugging you tightly in return."

Ronnie looked at me as if I were slightly peculiar and then said, "But Jesus is already here." To him, I was overlooking the obvious. The bone marrow went very smoothly.

Ronnie reminds me that all relationships, all imagination find their highest fulfillment in the presence of God who chose to take on flesh like ours and dwell among us. As Leanne Payne says:

> . . . to acknowledge the Presence of *the God who is really there* is actually a form of prayer, a way of praying always as the Scriptures exhort us to do. When we do this, the eyes and ears of our hearts are opened to receive the word he is always speaking.[2]

Adults are not without hope. Like Michelangelo, we can chisel away until we cut David loose. Like David, we can dance with Yahweh and catch fire. Like the children, we can blaze up in a single flame of such magnificence that neither life nor death nor anything else in all of creation can separate us from the love of God.

6

Converting a Contract
into a Covenant

❧

Love is responsibility of an I for a thou.
MARTIN BUBER

Dear Crumb Bunny,
You are in the last room in the row on the Bone Marrow
Unit and cannot see me when I come in. I pause, put on protective
shoe covers, chat with visitors. You hear my voice even before you
can see me. By the time I come into your view, you extend your little turtle neck, probing out of your shell. You pose and peek and
prance in anticipation. Dare I admit how flattered I am?

I watch you smile at me and know that it's not just that
you're special to me. I know that I am special to you. How can I
begin to describe my relationship to you? I cherish you as well. We
met because I am an expert on your rare disease. We all realize
today how important it was for you that I do know your disease so
well. But we've all grown beyond that day.

How can anyone meet you and just think about diseases,
facts, figures, lab results? You smile, you cry, you giggle (the most ordinary of human acts). Performed by you they are acts of rare beauty.

128

I provide you with my professional services, but a business contract does not adequately describe what we've been through the last year together. We will have to look further for proper words to describe our relationship, mine and thine.

Reading the morning paper, you would think that medical practice today is only business and politics. The situation seems utterly without hope.

The public thinks that the doctor-patient relationship isn't what it used to be. Doctors complain that the practice of medicine isn't what it used to be. At least there, we all agree. Things have changed.

There used to be something that made us happier than we are today. We all want the good from the good old days. Here physicians need not muse alone. There are others to share the speculation.

There was a time when Western medical ethics leaned regularly on theological concepts. Ethicist Paul Ramsey calls me back to "the Biblical norm of fidelity to covenant" when he interprets the practice of medicine as one such covenant.[1]

I like that word—*covenant*. But as I read the newspapers and listen to our elected representatives, all I hear are promises to negotiate for a better health-care *contract*. As I listen to the voices of the children, they remind me how the spirit of contracts and covenants so markedly differ. Ethicist William May says:

> Contracts are external; covenants are internal to the parties involved. . . . This discussion of contract and covenant, then, forces a return to the world that the biblical covenant presents, as it attempts to deal with the sting of disease, suffering and death.[2]

This understanding affords the opportunity to redefine the healing partnership between patient and physician. In the Bible there are many opportunities to examine the notion of covenant.

I like the story of Jacob and Laban because it tests the concept of covenant to its limits. The tension focuses on Rachel, Laban's daughter and Jacob's intended bride. If it were not for the bride, those two men would never have been talking to each other.

Two adults couldn't even agree which language to use when they assembled a group of stones as a "heap of witness" to their agreement. Each used his own language on his sign that marked the site, but they were willing to try because of a common goal that they shared.

Differences in personalities and conflicts of culture, belief, and sense of authority sometimes complicate the ability to live out the doctor-patient relationship as a covenant. We do, however, have a common goal as patients and doctors that makes it worthwhile to stretch toward each other.

José was three years old when a lump proved to be malignant. He received chemotherapy in an effort to avoid radical surgery. When a scan showed that the tumor was growing, we recommended surgery, but the family declined on the advice of a member of their church.

They based their hope on the words of this man who claimed the gift of prophecy that he had a "word from the Lord" that the boy was already healed. Surgery was not needed, he said.

We planned a conference with the parents and asked them to invite the "prophet" and their pastor. As we reviewed the medical facts for them, the church member looked defiant, avoiding eye contact with us, barely listening to our words. The parents gazed in pain and fear at their child. Their pastor listened carefully and asked our opinion about José's chances, with and without the surgery.

"Pastor, everyone in this room is on the same team. We all want José to be healed, and we all want to be sure that God is glorified however healing occurs. We'd like you to lead us in prayer for José."

We did not want to pressure the family to accept surgery or to reorient their theology. Our intent was to permit them to face a difficult medical decision, fully informed in a supportive environment where everyone was on their side. Even the "prophet" enthusiastically joined in the most unusual session that has ever been held in my office. We agreed to wait a week and perform another CAT scan. When that showed further tumor growth, surgery was scheduled.

By identifying that which we could share, we found seed for a covenant. In a covenantal relationship, there is the hope for win-win. This process is a form of "second opinion," calling on someone who shared the family's beliefs but could be objective. The pastor was in a better position than they or the church member to discern the difference between prophetic word and noble feeling.

Covenant-fidelity seeks a common ground that transcends individual or institutional authority and points to the perfect love that casts out fear. It does not require that the parties be in perfect agreement on all points, as in a contract.

But it is not always easy to think of the medical intercourse in these terms. Some doctors openly admit feelings of rage and frustration toward unappreciative patients. In an unusually frank essay, one physician expressed a fantasy that many have repressed:

> She tried to bite me. . . . When the people from the
> diet service came . . . she would either spit at them

or hurl a fork or knife their way. . . . My natural
urges were to choke her to death. In fact, it gave me
a lot of relief to fantasize how I would kill her. . . .
Still, every time she was admitted to our hospital,
Duchess got from all of us the best of modern medical care.[3]

Anyone who has practiced medicine knows a
Duchess. In talking about another "difficult" patient, physi-
cian-author Bernie Siegel comes closer to the notion of
covenant. He told a woman with breast cancer whose family
thought that she was crazy that he loved her and all that she
told him.[4]

It is not only difficult to think in a covenantal fashion,
but it is downright impossible in human terms. The very act
of writing about it reminds me how much help I need to carry
my part of a covenant forward. And how often I fail.

I sometimes write words like these at night and the
next day, come face-to-face with an "impossible" someone I
would rather avoid. But then I am reminded of Jesus' words:
"Just as you did it to one of the least of these who are members
of my family, you did it to me" (Matt. 25:40 NRSV).

Mother Teresa speaks of seeing a Person in a person.
With holy eyes, one might even see the Prince of Peace in a
Duchess. If it were Jesus himself who was my patient, just how
would I go through each step of a painful procedure? With
Jesus at my mercy, how much mercy would I show?

It is in relationship to Christ, his covenant with me,
and my covenant with him, that mercy guides my hand. With
a Person in my clinic, it is a safer place for children.

7

Big Joe and Little Joe

Schoolboys have no fear of facing life. They champ at
the bit.

ANTOINE SAINT-ÉXUPÉRY

Dear Crumb Bunny,

Parents are very important to babies. They can make all
the difference in the world to a child. Your mom cares about all the
babies and boys and girls she meets. She has a sensitivity to the crises
of these others, your spiritual brothers and sisters, and always
remembers to pray for them.

This morning Mom asked me about one boy because of her
special concern for him. Two floors away on another hospital ward,
he had just died. His sudden death was a surprise to us. Somehow,
a mother's praying heart had known.

You are your mother's darling and mine as well. Somehow
I think that you know that. Doctors aren't supposed to have preferences, but no one begrudges me my special relationship with you.

I brag about you almost more than your mother does.
Everyone has to put up with me telling Crumb Bunny stories and
my latest dream for you. The teenage patients listen and grin

133

knowingly. They're partial to babies—and dreams too. Then they add, more solemnly, "I can understand for myself. I've lived. But the babies get to me. They haven't ever lived." They love you, too, and hope and pray for your recovery.

Someday I would like to introduce you to some of my other favorites. You may crowd out the room, but I think you would all like each other a lot.

❧

It was a shock to open the newspaper and see his picture. To be sure, he must have been proud to be pictured with his ice hockey team. He had hemophilia, and we had advised against contact sports.

He was nine years old then and my concerns were for hemorrhage. But his parents were committed to normalizing his life, so they infused him with concentrate and allowed him to live. They have never regretted that decision.

His mother listened very carefully when several years later we explained about the newly discovered problem of contamination of blood factor concentrate for hemophilia by the agent that caused AIDS. HIV had not yet been discovered, nor was there yet a blood test to determine if a blood donor was infected.

In that era, concentrates offered a convenient way for hemophiliacs to treat themselves at home. But since they concentrated the blood of many, many donors, they also posed the greatest risk from AIDS. When the blood of a single infected donor was pooled with five hundred others, it was as if all five hundred had been infected.

That year, our best advice was to surrender the freedom that the concentrates of many blood donors provided. Old fashioned "cryo" wasn't as convenient, but it used fewer donors to achieve the same dose. Joe made the switch to cryo.

Despite these precautions, eventually Big Joe tested positive for HIV. Four years later, two weeks before Thanksgiving, I was standing by his bed in our Pediatric Intensive Care Unit. A respirator was breathing for him and he was fighting for his life. That was the day he became "Big Joe."

In the bed next to him was another of our team's patients who had just reached the age at which Big Joe had played ice hockey. "Little Joe" had been diagnosed with a rare form of cancer in the same year that we learned that Big Joe was HIV-positive.

Despite all our efforts, the cancer kept coming back in his lungs. Now his chest was filling up with fluid, and he could not breathe without help. There was room for no more radiation, and we knew of no other effective treatment. Chest tubes could only drain the fluid for a little while before it would reaccumulate.

Our pediatric surgeons were willing to try to strip off the lining around the lung that seemed to be "weeping" in response to the cancer, but the procedure was risky. He might not come through the operation at all. Even if he did, he might not be able to breathe on his own and would forever need the use of a respirator.

A brave young boy had made his own decision to try the operation and, characteristically, he survived it. Now our Little Joe, still on a respirator, was bedded down next to our Big Joe. The holiday season did not seem to be off to a promising start.

I have great respect for the special pediatricians who supervise our PICU. In our hospital jargon they are known as "intensivists," and that aptly describes their work. A member of this team approached Big Joe's parents to tell them his grim interpretation of the current findings. The doctor gently probed their feelings about heroic measures and asked if Joe had ever indicated his own preferences.

His mom shook her head when I made my rounds. "This may sound dumb, but I don't think he's going to die this time. He's going to survive this infection. This isn't going to be the one that gets him." There was nothing I could read on the chart to support her optimism. My colleague was right to assume that he might die.

In the next bed it was apparent that recovery from the anesthesia did not mean recovery of independent breathing. Little Joe was still on a respirator and plans were considered to place a "trach" (breathing tube) in his windpipe. There were no sudden success stories in the PICU for our team, no sagas of dramatic recovery.

It was getting tougher and tougher to make those visits to the PICU. One runs out of words and finds oneself fussing with bedside charts and numbers, sharing data rather than feelings. Data don't bite quite so badly.

When you run out of words, it feels safer to round with a team, swooping down on patient and family with your roving band of residents and students. As we approached Big Joe's bed, his mom was reading a small plastic card in front of her. When she saw us coming, she quickly stuffed it in her pocket.

When the others moved on to Little Joe, I lingered behind. "What was that you stuffed in your pocket to hide when we came in?" She blushed and produced a card with a prayer printed on it. "Don't you dare hide anything like that ever again! It's not an either/or matter, medicine and faith."

Little Joe had his trach in place and was not yet able to speak. This made a little man of few words very, very gabby. Except that he was without a voice. So he kept mouthing words and pointing. On his tray table were plaster penguins that he was painting. It was apparent that our Child Life Program had conquered this sanctum sanctorum of technological medicine.

By Thanksgiving Day, even his cousins had invaded. A room next to the PICU became their workshop for the creation of tiny gingerbread houses out of graham crackers, icing, gum drops, and whatever else caught the young architects' fancy. Countertops that are ordinarily littered with ribbons of EKG tracings spewed out by the cardiac monitors were tidied up to become the display case for dozens of these little beauties.

Little Joe's pointing finger became his voice. As nurses and doctors came in, he indicated that each should choose a gingerbread house to take home. It was an honor to carry my new treasure off to my office, happy that Little Joe could divert himself but concerned whether he would ever leave the PICU and the hospital alive.

Big Joe held his own, but there was extensive damage to vital organs. He remained sedated so that he would not fight the ventilator that supported his life. His parents were most often by his bedside, but sometimes I would find his dad visiting with Little Joe and his parents. They had more than a common name and common doctors that bound them together.

Eventually Big Joe woke up as well and both of our Joes were transferred to a regular floor to complete their convalescence. Big Joe was the first to make it home. Although he had lost weight during the illness and required a wheelchair until he regained strength, he made a remarkable recovery.

Little Joe remained with us because of the powerful ventilator that he required. At Christmas his room filled with gifts and new craft projects. Little Joe lived on and began to think about going home even if it was to die. Somehow, the impossible became possible. He and his breathing machine moved home where his hospital-based doctors and nurses continued to visit and supervise his care.

Big Joe recovered enough to travel to Europe and return to college. A year later, he is as handsome as ever and full of plans for the future. I saw Big Joe's mom in our clinic once, writing a letter while she waited for her son.

She was carefully choosing her words to write to a PICU doctor. During the crisis, he had asked her about withdrawal of life support. "I want to be constructive," she said, "so that the doctors will learn from the experience how important faith and hope are in determining what happens to these kids. I mostly want to thank him for his excellent care and update him on all that Joe has been able to accomplish during the last year."

I commended her for her intentions and reflected, "Here it is a year later. Who would ever have believed that both Big Joe and Little Joe would still be with us?"

"Little Joe?" she asked with great surprise. "I had no idea that he was still alive. I was always afraid to ask."

"O ye of little faith!" I teased in return.

I look today at Big Joe, who is still HIV-positive, and Little Joe, who still has cancer, and I know what the statistics say. But for a quarter of a century I have been quoting statistics and learning that the human spirit is stronger than any probability. Statistically, neither Big Joe nor Little Joe should be here today. So with them and their parents, I continue to hope.

8

Hearts Unfolding

~~~~~~~

God of glory, Lord of love, hearts unfold like flowers
before thee, opening to the sun above.

<div align="right">HENRY VAN DYKE</div>

Dear Crumb Bunny,

You are like a flower, little princess. You sit in your laminar air-flow room flirting with me and cooing at your nurses. You
love your little tape recorder and keep listening to the words: "Jesus
wants me for a sunbeam to shine for him today." You don't just
shine, Baby. You dazzle.

There was a reason I ordered all those baby IQ tests before
you were admitted to the Bone Marrow Transplant Unit. I wanted to
see if the histiocytes that we found in your brain and spinal fluid had
caused any damage. The psychologist called you "precocious" in some
areas he tested. He must have offered you a tape recorder to play with.

Much of what we do in testing babies is to see how you
respond to games we adults design. We don't seem much interested
or very talented in testing your spiritual development. Even if we
were interested, we would probably invent tests to see whether you
babies have learned from adults about God and such.

I look at you and feel you embrace me with your smile. I wonder how you would design a test to measure my spiritual IQ?

Some time ago, I visited a church in a community where no one knows me. A mother and three children sat down in the pew in front of me, and an eight-year-old carrot-topped girl turned around to greet me. "My father's in the hospital," she declared. "It's his kidney."

I was stunned at first because she had no way of knowing that I was a doctor. Her concern and worry were unmistakable. So I recovered myself and said to her, "Then we'll have to pray for him." She nodded with redheaded vigor.

The worship service opened with announcements that included the sharing of the sort of concern that was burdening this young child. When the pastor asked if anyone had anything to share, her hand shot up. Just as quickly, her mother and older brother grabbed her arm and lowered it.

The announcements came and went without her concerns for her daddy being raised to her community of faith. The next part of the service was the greeting. As quickly as the pastor invited worshipers to greet each other, my little friend sprang into the aisle, with her hand extended. She covered at least ten rows in the time available, greeting each worshiper with, "My father's in the hospital. It's his kidney."

Of all of the worshipers, only this tender young flower was willing to become vulnerable as she spread her petals and exposed her delicate inner structure in response to heavenly sunshine.

As adults, we seem to have limited expectations of children. We hardly expect them to be *our* teachers. Two millenia ago, when young children saw Jesus and cried out to him in the temple, the adults present became angry. Jesus' response to them was this: "Out of the mouths of infants and nursing babes you [meaning God] have prepared praise for yourself."

I've thought about my little redhead often when I've been in my medical office seeing patients. There are close analogies between her holy vulnerability and that of my patients. In the family of faith, she found a reason to hope. I wonder why her mother did not share her own concern publicly with her faith-family. Surely it was heavy upon her own heart.

Her mother's silence was typical adult behavior. One reason I enjoy my practice with children is their ability to express themselves. And express themselves they will when adults permit. I was touched a few weeks ago in my own church when the joys and concerns were shared.

A little girl from my own home church was diagnosed with leukemia. A school chum of hers stood up in our worship service and asked for prayer for her friend. I tried to imagine how the congregation would have reacted had the pastor or another adult shared the news with us. We were touched not only by the child's illness but by the faithfulness of her little friend.

Out of the mouths of babes. Had God prepared that young girl to prepare us? These were the words of hope that came to my mind, the very words of Scripture on which that part of our liturgy is based:

> Are any among you suffering? They should pray. Are any cheerful? They should sing songs of praise. Are any among you sick? ... Pray for one another, so that you may be healed. The prayer of the righteous is powerful and effective. (James 5:13–14, 16 NRSV)

Are you really surprised that children can teach us so much? A baby's smile encourages us to unfold our stiff adult petals faster than any reasoned lecture on honesty and transparency can. My little Crumb Bunny helped me and everyone else who visited her in the Bone Marrow Unit to shed our protective layers when she laughed at a silly game we played. She was learning new words in those days. As her vocabulary was expanding, we competed to see whose name would be next after *dada* and *mama*. The baby had always heard me called "Dr. Komp," but the letter *K* is a late sound to be mastered by a baby. Some informality seemed necessary, so I capitalized on her familiarity with *hi*. Our daily ritual was "Hi, Di!"

Nurse Angie was not about to be outwitted. The baby woke up each morning in her life island, calling to any of the nurses standing near the desk. *Aaaaaaah.* Angie insisted that she was saying *Aaaaaangie.*

Then there was the all-important Hanne who would be the one to fly to London to pick up the donated bone marrow. The baby had a standard answer to all requests, common to her age: No, more often heard as "nah." Hanne picked up her negation, *nah*, repeated it at least once an hour. "Can't you tell?" said Hanne with chin held high. "She's saying (Han)ne."

This was our daily game in which our little co-conspirator delighted. *My name first! Return my love with my name on your lips. I would give anything in the world to hear you, blessed child, say my name.*

They didn't teach me to play such games in medical school, but things are changing. When I was a student, there was no place for a future doctor who might weep. There is evidence of hope, even in the "gross" anatomy lab:

> Nervous students in surgical gloves and aprons . . .
> lined up alongside steel tables where cadavers lay
> ready for dissection. Instead of feeling pressured to
> maintain a stoic composure, these first-year med-
> ical students were encouraged not to suppress their
> emotions but to cry, laugh, faint, or leave the room
> if they wanted to. None did, but many said they

appreciated the "permission" to do so. . . . "We try to tell them it's okay to feel weird, upset about what they're doing."[1]

At Dartmouth Medical School, former Surgeon General C. Everett Koop has been the catalyst for change toward a different style of mentoring. He and his colleagues hope to inspire future physicians to be more human in their relationships with patients. Such changes in medical education are overdo and might just help resuscitate our mortally ill health-care system.

What would happen to the health care of adults if one highly trained doctor and two super-specialized nurses spent as much time unfolding their hearts the way Angie and Hanne and I did to Crumb Bunny? Could just *one* doctor plead with just *one* adult patient, *Please show me that you love me. Say my name first?* Don't laugh at me. I'm entitled to my dreams. And so are you.

143

9

The Apple Doll House Parables

No, it was to shame the wise that God chose what is
foolish by human reckoning.

1 CORINTHIANS 1:27 (JB)

Dear Crumb Bunny,

I look at Mom looking at you as we talk and I know that
you are loved and accepted. Her idea of a perfect Crumb Bunny is
just the way you are, and will be.

Someday you'll meet my friend Ruth. Her son, Donny,
died ten years ago, but I still think of him in the present tense. Ruth
knows how to value special people. After Donny's death, she went
to work at the Apple Doll House.

At the Apple Doll House, you could meet some of the
weakest and most vulnerable members of our community. But
there, they could come and work and hold their heads high.

I watch you, my little love, and note that you are one of the
wise ones. I know that when you grow up you will have a heart for
God's most fragile creatures.

We have no idea yet what causes most cases of cancer in children. For most it happens without warning. Not so for some of my most special patients, children with Down's syndrome. Their abnormal chromosome can lead to cancer as well as birth defects. Morris West calls them the "clowns of God."

Leukemia is their most common malignancy, but other tumors happen as well. What distinguishes the Down's child with cancer from others in my practice is that their parents come so well-prepared. Oddly enough, I find that these special children have also been my most valued teachers.

During my training, we were advised to recommend institutionalization to families of retarded children. Now most of them grow up in their families, supported by regional centers. And some of these regional centers are extra, extra special.

The Apple Doll House is closed now as a restaurant but its building is used for other worthy purposes. It was in this restaurant that some of my fondest memories took shape.

I had a phone call one day from a man who identified himself as a computer specialist. His teenage son with Down's syndrome had undergone surgery for cancer and they hoped to find the right doctor to coordinate his further care.

His surgeon thought that an adult oncologist would be appropriate since it was an adult-type tumor in an adult-sized person. But Down's syndrome had complicated Rodd's entire life. His parents could not believe that their son should be managed like the average adult.

Rodd's father used his own expertise to shop among pediatricians for the "right" doctor. Although he had never sought someone with special expertise in cancer in Down's syndrome, my name kept appearing on other computer programs he used. "But who told you about my special interest in Down's syndrome?" I asked. I had never published anything on the subject. My "expertise" is defined by my love for God's special clowns.

"Then we really were 'sent' to you!" he replied. "I didn't even know that."

Rodd's tumor is cured, but we keep in frequent touch because of mutual respect and unrivaled fun. He would even agree to a barium enema if I curtsied properly and called him "Your Lordship."

Rodd is witty, active, and proud and would dance me off my feet at his birthday parties if I didn't plead middle age and propose a younger partner. Praise the Lord for amazing Grace. His girlfriend, who also has Down's syndrome, can dance all night.

We last met at Apple Doll House Restaurant. This time, he was my guest. Mary Kate, the senior hostess, came to take our orders. As His Lordship perused the menu, he sneaked a glimpse of this wondrous creature out of the corner of his eye. All the dining-room staff that day were adults with Down's syndrome, and Rodd thought he was in heaven when he saw who was running the place.

As Mary Kate glided away from the table with our orders, Rodd permitted himself a cautious sideward glance then returned his attention to us. He shook his head contemplatively and said, "Stunning woman!"

Mary Kate returned with our desserts and the check. As we were leaving the Apple Doll House, his mother asked, "Rodd, what do you think of this place?" He looked around him and said wistfully but clearly, "It's wonderful to see so many handicapped people."

Do you think it's wonderful when you see many handicapped people? We, the clever, are often the ones who are lacking in ability. And definitely lacking in imagination. One young man I know with severely impaired speech is in love. His sweetheart, who is deaf, taught him sign language, and she "hears" only the beautiful fluency of his hands.

Because of a major birth defect, Harold Wilke lacks the hands to execute sign language, but he has perhaps the most talented toes in Christendom. Dr. Karl Menninger quotes Rev. Wilke: "I can't shake hands with you . . . I never had hands . . . I was expected by my parents to do everything my brothers did, and I learned alternative ways—toes instead of fingers."[1]

Do you hope to see many handicapped, special people in the course of your day? Not if you are typical of our society. It is not only society and the health-care system that may fail our handicapped citizens. Historically, the religious community has not done much better. Reverend Wilke would not always have been considered candidate material for ordained ministry.

Do you, like Rodd, find it "wonderful"? Or, is your first impulse to run? Sometimes we run in hospitals, and even in houses of worship. We may not exclude the mentally and physically handicapped by policy, but we, the clever, seem chronically lacking in imagination. Without holy imagination and the gift to include, we are not a people of hope.

We can respond to what is weak and foolish, common and contemptible by human reckoning. If we examine our impulses and stop running, we can become a caring society. We *are* a healing community when we use a thousand tongues and fingers and toes to repeat God's finest whispers.

10

A Matter of Life and Death

Life is serious all the time, but living cannot be . . . You
may have all the solemnity you wish in your neckties,
but in anything important (such as sex, death, and religion), you must have mirth or you will have madness.

G. K. CHESTERTON

Dear Crumb Bunny,

A bone-marrow ward is a place to think about life and
death. All the patients are here because they desperately want to
live, but not everyone will walk out through the door. No one
knows better than the doctors and nurses who work here what it
means to contemplate life and death in the same thought, capture
their essence in the same breath.

You babies who have come here as patients have taught us
much. You know what it means to be vulnerable but trusting,
dependent but not depressed. That's a hard lesson but a necessary
one for adults to learn.

There are older kids and adults in this hospital who must
sometimes wear a diaper. But unlike you, they weep when they soil,

*and someone else must come to change them. They are very proud
people, as Jesus knew.*

*The Christian story says that God partook in our experi-
ence, shared that tension on the edge of life and death. God was dia-
pered in Bethlehem, learned to say Abba in a carpenter's shop. And
when he had profound lessons to share with adults about life and
death and pride, he pointed to someone like a little Crumb Bunny.*

You are a teacher, little one, with a message for us all.

When a child comes to our wards with the diagnosis
of cancer, someone may ask whether the patient realizes that
he is dying. But cancer is a word, not a sentence. Cancer is easier to heal than a morbid fear of cancer.

Vulnerable children have taught me not to fear fear
itself. I've learned from the children and their parents that not
all fear of cancer should be avoided.

Fear can alert us to danger. It only becomes noxious
when our response, our fear of our fear, prevents us from moving in life-affirming ways.

If I feel a lump in my breast and fear that it is cancer, I
can move in one of two directions. Fear can move me to a doctor for early diagnosis and treatment. Or fear can lead me to pro-
crastinate and deny what seems to be. Fear can propose fantasies
and invite inertia. But if fear compels me to act, fear is my friend.

"I have a terminal illness," says Peter Kreeft, author of
Love Is Stronger Than Death. "You are invited to read for the
same reason.... Life is always fatal. No one gets out of it
alive."[1] Someone with cancer is no more "terminal" than the
rest of us. Nor are they to be subjected to pitiful pity.

In the adult world, one of the greatest impediments to
conquering cancer is the delay in diagnosis. A false kind of
hope spins tales to the psyche. This is rarely seen with children. The typical child I see for cancer is brought to a doctor

the same day the first symptom is recognized. This is an important reason that we have made so much progress in their care.

The Big C. The greatest fear. Such toxic fear takes on magical qualities in some of the most rational, nonmagical thinkers I know. I see this force at work when I meet people for the first time and the conversation turns to the usual small talk. When I say that I am a pediatric oncologist, I wait for the automatic small step backward, away from me. My patients know this fear as well, that our proximity might hex those who come near them or someone they love. This is magical thinking, but popular even among the educated.

Once when I was shopping, an almost-voiceless friend sought my medical opinion. She showed me an antibiotic that remained on her bathroom shelf after a previous illness. She was suffering from laryngitis and wondered if these capsules would help. This particular medicine does nothing for viral infections and can have undesirable side effects. I recommended that she not take them.

Another customer overheard our conversation. He had no idea who I was but thought that he certainly had more to offer than a middle-aged woman in shorts and a T-shirt. "That antibiotic can do you no harm," he disagreed without being consulted, and my friend asked him if he was a doctor. No, he wasn't. He was a dentist.

She thought she should clarify who I was. "That woman with whom I was talking, she's a medical doctor. She's an oncologist."

"Oncologist!" he exclaimed, assuming I was out of earshot. "Do you know what that means? All her patients are terminal. Why, that's pitiful!"

We tend to divide life from death, living from dying, as if they happen to two different sets of people. With the dying we place all those with cancer. Another personal experience reminds me how difficult it is to think of life and death at the same time.

I was leading a seminar for physicians and clergy who came together to explore their common interest in physical and spiritual wholeness. A hospital chaplain who attended expressed his desire to see better communication with his medical friends. "The way I see it," he explained, "doctors should let the clergy know when someone is dying. That is where your job ends and ours begins." His statement captured my full attention. He startled me.

Some physicians flee the bedsides of the dying as if we ourselves are not safe. When we do, we leave a gap, forsaking the sufferer. It was this gap that the chaplain saw. But did he not leave another gap in its place? I would have thought that he, like Jesus, might have something to offer the living as well as the dying. As I understand it, the Christian gospel, which the chaplain was ordained to proclaim, is *good* news.

The chaplain saw his job and mine as serial rather than parallel, independent rather than interdigitating. My responsibility and the hope that I can bring does not end with the last prescription. To keep the covenant, I must address my own fear of cancer, my own fear of death, and move back to the bedside. "Til death us do part," a covenantal promise, would make a more appropriate summary statement for a doctor-patient relationship. And that is not bad news at all. It is a reason to hope.

"Peace I leave with you," said Jesus. "My peace I give to you. I do not give to you as the world gives. Do not let your hearts be troubled, and do not let them be afraid" (John 14:27, NRSV). This peace he speaks of is more than the absence of fear. It is a gift from Christ for those who make the choice. "*Do not let your hearts be troubled*" is a command, not a suggestion. It is a choice we can all make. And that is good news indeed.

To participate in the healing of others, we ourselves must do something about our own wounds. We need to start with our ideas about life. For some bizarre reason, we think that we are already experts about life and that it is only death that holds the unknown. The grim statistics on failed marriage, unwanted pregnancy, dysfunctional families, and social despair cry out that we have much as a society to learn about life. We need valid reasons to hope.

Since the publication of Elisabeth Kübler-Ross's book, *On Death and Dying*, some have said that death has come "out of the closet."[2] Dying seems to have found a way to separate itself from living, to take on, so to speak, a life of its own.

We can learn much about life, healing, and hope from those who work with the dying. Shiela Cassidy, a British hospice physician, says that she has a "very expensive ringside seat at the fight" but concludes:

> We have a duty to report back the truth of what we see: that the facts are friendly; that the blind see, the lame walk, the lepers are cleansed, and the good news is proclaimed to the poor—that the kingdom of God is among us, and that herein lies our hope.[3]

A few years ago a close friend of mine struggled with widespread cancer. On a drive to Boston following a chemotherapy cycle, we made many emergency stops. Each time Ginnie returned, she looked a bit wearier and a lot paler. I would resume driving without comment, until the next stop.

One time, she got back in the car and looked up at me with a mischievous little-child grin to say, "This is going to sound very corny. The Big C isn't cancer. The Big C is Christ." For her, no disease would be allowed to take on power in her life. Cancer would not have the last laugh. In choosing to make Christ the center of her life, Ginnie could face cancer, chemotherapy, and even death itself unbowed. In making that choice, she was healed of the fear of cancer and the fear of death.

Not many months later, the tumors were growing in her body and it was time to invite hospice into her home. She called me at work many times to say, "Tell your patients, hospice is about life."

Christ is the Big C. Hospice is life. These statements do not ignore mortality. They simply put cancer and death into their proper perspective. In Christ and with hospice, Ginnie found that she would never be alone or abandoned. She was free to live and laugh.

In some Greek communities, Christians gather the day after Easter to tell each other jokes, honoring God's greatest joke that took place on Easter morn.[4] But the healing property of humor is lost if we don't get the joke and fail to understand the punch line.

> When this perishable body puts on imperishability, and this mortal body puts on immortality, then the saying that is written will be fulfilled: "Death has been swallowed up in victory." (1 Cor. 15:54 NRSV)

A friend told me that in his family the members whose lives have been touched by cancer have the best sense of humor. I can understand this. It is children with cancer who taught me hilarity, to risk laughing when the world might dictate tears. One child tells me that it is when he hears me laugh that he knows he has hope.

In reaching my hand to the plastic window that separates Crumb Bunny from me, I delight in her delight of me. We do not let our hearts be troubled. We both have a terminal illness, she and I, but we have a reason to hope. *Where, O death, is your victory? Where, O death, is your sting?* She giggles and I giggle, sharing our Easter hilarity. We both understand God's greatest joke.

11

Risen with Healing
in His Wings

Life and light to all he brings, risen with healing in his wings.
CHARLES WESLEY

Dear Crumb Bunny,

The statistics say that you have no hope to survive. You will die, they say, that none of my medical miracles will avail. Because of those statistics, I am reaching beyond what is familiar, and the reach is wider than some suspect.

Does Dr. Grandma pray for you to be healed? Baby, you had better believe it. Someone very wise summarized our journey together, yours and mine: "Work as if everything depends on you and pray as if everything depends on God." Your doctor is into combined modality therapy.

Some people believe there never were any miracles. Other people believe that there were only miracles during the time that the Bible was being written and then they stopped. Still others think that God only works miracles independent of medical intervention. The *arguments are without end. Personally, I think some of those people are well-meaning but a little bit confused.*

I have lived too long and seen too much to tie you up in tidy intellectual knots. Because I hope, my princess, I work and pray for you to be healed.

❧

It was one of those collegial but challenging conferences where physicians of different disciplines exchanged ideas on difficult tumor cases. The case at hand was that of a baby who had broken all the rules.

"Are you sure you had the right diagnosis?" asked the radiotherapist of the pathologist. "I've never seen this particular tumor respond that way. You must be wrong."

"No, I'm not wrong!" responded the somewhat indignant pathologist. "I know that tumor when I see it."

"Well, maybe you want to look at it again."

"Looking at it again isn't going to change the diagnosis!'"

The radiation therapist looked elsewhere for an explanation of the unexplainable and turned to the chemotherapist managing the case. "That chemotherapy must have done the job."

"Don't look over here for the explanation," said her chemotherapist. "We only used a radio-sensitizing dose. Besides, the tumor was growing through the last course of different drugs. Are you sure it wasn't the radiation therapy that did the job?"

"No way. This tumor has never gone away like that before." He turned half-joking to the radiologist who had interpreted the scans. "Are you sure those are the right films?"

"Yes, they're the right X-rays! You can tell from the comparison to the old ones that it's the same child. Only the tumor is gone."

"It doesn't make sense," the radiation therapist kept repeating.

The minutes of that conference simply reflected the lack of a known medical explanation for the disappearance of the tumor. The medical minutes did not reflect other activities on her behalf. Teams from a local church fasted and prayed daily for Bethany, two by two. Many other family friends prayed for her tumor to go away.

These days if the word *healing* is used in conjunction with health, it is most often interpreted to reflect some activity other than medical practice. Several years ago, I had lunch at a Trappist monastery with a former brother of that community. Before lunch we attended a service with the brothers and other guests. During the prayers of the people, my companion asked prayer for, "My friend Di, and her ministry of healing."

At lunch, several fellow-guests asked me about my "ministry of healing." They were shocked to learn that I am a medical doctor. They did not expect a "healer" to be a medical doctor. Personally, I am not comfortable with the term "healer" for any human person. There is a sign over a mission hospital that summarizes it all for me: *We treat; Jesus heals*. I simply cooperate. I am part of God's combined modality team.

"I have a brilliant idea about how to reduce Francesca's side effects," I proudly announced to a mother. For months her child's blood counts had dipped dangerously low, and now I had an idea how to avoid that problem.

"You and your brilliant ideas!" sassed her mother in return. "Some of us parents have been talking. We pray and then you get your brilliant ideas. Just don't take all the credit!" Her blood counts never reached the danger level again.

❦

"My miracle man!" was the greeting of a cardiologist who brought Mike back from the jaws of death when he removed a clot from a vital coronary artery. Days earlier when I joined my friend's family and pastor in the coronary care unit, the "miracle man" was in shock and dying. As the medical team was preparing to take Mike for a final attempt to save his life, we were praying (against the odds) for his recovery.

A nurse moved toward our circle, but the doctor held her back. "Don't interrupt them," he said quietly. "They are praying." The same nurse called my office an hour later to say, "It's a miracle. He's out of shock. We can hardly believe it."

❦

The families I just described all have an active concept of healing. But what would they think if they consulted me in my medical office and I said, "I am sure that I can heal your child?" They would probably run out the door to find themselves a "real" doctor. Patients expect a different vocabulary from a medical specialist who fits squarely within traditional Western medicine. But the three families I described have not placed all their hope in imperfect scientists.

❦

What if Mike has another heart attack? How will Francesca's family react if their daughter's future life is not one of perfect health? What will all those praying people think if Bethany has only a remission and not a cure of her malignancy?

I worry about people whose faith is based on their ability to get God to perform on command. The families I describe and their friends are not such people. They have met other faithful families whose loved ones have not survived and have seen the healing presence of God in their lives despite their losses. The world is a richer place for the journeys that they've all traveled.

The adults in these stories have come into a relationship with God that cannot be changed by subsequent medical events. The whole work of God is displayed in their lives for they themselves have been healed.

Are these stories miracles of divine healing or miracles of modern medical science? All of these families involved were convinced of a spiritual element in their loved one's improved health. But they were equally convinced of the value of modern medical care and continue to comply diligently with all orthodox medical recommendations. For them it is not an either/or matter. Neither is it for me.

Never far behind the question about divine healing are questions about divine reasons why children suffer. Jesus was asked one day by his own friends. "Who sinned, this man or his parents, that he was born blind?" (John 9:2 NIV). His answer was quite simple: "Neither this man nor his parents sinned." Parents tormented by imagined guilt think that the answer to their offspring's cancer is who. And the "who" must be themselves.

Jesus took clay from the earth, mixed it with his own saliva and put it on the man's eyes "so that the work of God might be displayed in his life" (John 9:3 NIV). Jesus converted *why* and *who* into *what*. I feel compelled to do the same.

"Do you believe in healing?" asks a young mother, and I know in my heart that she is not asking if I believe that the chemotherapy I just gave her baby will work. And if she is anything like other mothers, she is wondering why her baby got cancer—if she herself is in some way responsible.

I move past the why and the who and consider what I can offer the young woman's baby, not only from modern medicine but also from God. I know that if that medical treatment has not worked for all such infants, it has worked for many. I cannot hold back from recommending it for her son because it hasn't worked every time. The same holds true for prayer.

I will not hold back from asking for God's personal healing touch on her baby because other children have died despite earnest prayer. I have seen the unexpected too often. Nor will I ask God to make a clear distinction between my work and his. My work is his as well. But I suggest to Naomi that she put every facet of her life, not just the baby's tumor, in God's hands and that she invite her husband to join her as well.

As a physician, I will work as hard as I can in a profession with an honorable history. As a Christian, I will also pray as hard as I can in a religious tradition that I also hold to be honorable. Children need to be healed. So do the rest of us.

12

Beauty by Proximity

⚡

To keep beauty in its place is to make all things beautiful.
GEORGE SANTAYANA

Dear Crumb Bunny,
From your life island you smile invitingly, pleased when I come up against your window. You reach your pudgy little hand toward me and play your tape recorder. When the song is complete, you remove the cassette and unravel the tape. Then you laugh and look to Mom for approval.

Since the day that you started your treatment, you have been a very busy baby. Your hospital visit days were packed full. You ate and slept and flirted and modeled one of your many prissy little dresses.

I think you were born knowing you were a girl-baby. Your idea of a wardrobe is a frock a day. Have you ever worn the same outfit twice? I think you will be a bit vain when you grow up. Vain, perhaps, but very beautiful. Since you're a baby, we'll allow such righteous vanity!

Don't stop there when it comes to beauty, little friend. You come from a family of heart-beautiful people.

Learn what you can from staying close to Mom and Dad.
Then, my dear, you will truly be beautiful.

"You know, it's all in the make-up and lighting,'" the photographer offered as he tried to get his subject to relax for the camera. "You wouldn't even recognize most of the top models outside the studio." *Life* magazine had sent him to my home to transform a middle-aged academic into proper pictorial material.

I adjusted the collar of my dress to hide my second chin. "Don't worry about that," he encouraged. "I can take care of that." He was visibly relieved when my Yorkshire Terrier climbed into my lap. To the photographer's delight, Ashley started posing without being coached. "He's great!" he exclaimed and then carefully added, "You're not bad yourself."

The conversation ultimately turned to world-famous beauties. Most beautiful women make it hard for the other people in the same photo, devastating them by comparison. Princess Di, on the other hand, is not only beautiful herself, she makes other people look good as well. Her shy smile enhances how we perceive her companions. When she weeps, we see her companions naked, as they are without her presence.

Finally the photographer called, "It's a wrap!" and he indicated to his assistant which film rolls to mark with a star. These were the shots when the dog was at his best. Hopefully, Doctor Di had been suitably beautified by proximity.

This "beauty by proximity" is something I see each day in a clinic where bodies have been seemingly ravaged by disease and treatment. We used to have a sign in our clinic that said, "Bald is beautiful." And years ago another one said, "Thank you, Kojak." Today it's Michael Jordan we adore.

One of my four-year-olds said years ago, "It's what's on a person's inside that counts." She knew how beautiful she was and allowed you (if you were nice) to stroke her shiny bald head.

When the head must be covered, fashionable headgear is a popular alternative for the kids. One mother designed a railroad engineer's cap for her daughter out of a patchwork of leftover fabric. Soon, every girl in her school had to have a similar hat. In that school, Barbara set the new standard for beauty. Long after she completed her treatment and her hair grew back, she and her classmates were still wearing those caps.

The more time I spend with these children, the more contagious I find their beauty of the heart. There is one advantage to not having hair—their eyes draw our own and become their focal feature.

The eyes are invariably eloquent, mirroring the heart and health. After their hair grows back, I still find myself drawn first to their eyes. For patients, the doctors' eyes are important as well. It is to our eyes rather than our words that they turn to measure truth and hope.

Years ago I explained to a father that his four-year-old daughter would lose her hair. He asked if it would not be better to leave her leukemia untreated and simply let her die. Fifteen years later, she is a college student, cured of leukemia. I still see her eyes first and don't even notice her hair.

Oh, I know it is there, fully regrown, but for the life of me I would be hard-pressed to tell you what color it is. But her eyes, yes, her eyes are an impish blue, framed by long lustrous lashes. She looks boldly into my eyes, challenging me to explore her very soul.

Many physicians freely admit that they choose other areas of medicine because they do not want to be near the suffering of children. They worry if a career in pediatrics would engender constant concern for the welfare of their own families. They know that even children suffer and die. Sometimes they fear the consequences, should one little one look deep into their very soul.

Similarly, many young physicians assume that our oncology clinic must be the most depressing assignment that they will face during their training. Most of them are unprepared for the opportunities for self-beautification. Some kids are more direct than others in their efforts to improve upon the rough-hewn humans who are their caregivers. I warned an intern one day before we knocked to see if Marnie was ready for examination.

"How many times do I have to tell you!" Marnie said, sadly shaking her head at me in disapproval. "You use the wrong shade of 'Loving Care.' You can still see the gray. There's absolutely no reason for you to look this old."

"But Marnie, I *am* this old. Middle age isn't a disease," I lamely protested.

"You don't act old. Why should you look so old?" retorted this pert teenager. "Gray hair is for people like my mother."

"Motherhood isn't a disease either. Besides, I'm older than your mother."

"Next time I come back, I expect to see no visible gray hair." That was her final pronouncement. It is a fearful thing to fall into the hands of a living teenager.

Marnie herself is a beautiful girl who was coping creatively with the changes that chemotherapy imposed upon her young body. A carefully chosen wig disguises her baldness, and skillfully applied makeup enhances her lovely features. She is impatient with me when I wear my trifocals instead of contact lenses and pay more attention to my paperwork than to my appearance.

This self-assured young woman who cheerfully greets everyone when she walks into the chemotherapy room is far different from the teenager I met months ago. The diagnosis of cancer and its aftermath accentuated a sadness she had experienced for many years. Ironically, it was in this oncology clinic that she herself was bequeathed beauty by proximity.

Competent care involves more than the application of scientific principles and protocols. We were fortunate to have a nursing assistant as a member of our team who brought out the beauty of all those whose lives she touched. Esther cradled many a teenager as we performed bone marrow aspirates and spinal taps as part of their treatment.

"You're my baby," I would hear her purr. "If I hold you, nothing bad can happen to you." When Marnie needed to share something painful with me, she confided in me from the safety of Esther's arms.

When we first met Marnie, she had no idea how beautiful a person she was on the inside. Coached by Esther, she learned her own worth. That beauty now radiates from the inside and touches all members of our extended family who have the good fortune to meet her.

Am I contradicting myself to simultaneously speak of physical and inner beauty? Not at all. For young women with cancer like Marnie, we must sometimes restore the sense of physical beauty before the beauty of the heart can shine through. Programs such as "Look Good/Feel Better" through the American Cancer Society recreate beauty from ashes, self-esteem from side effects. More than most women, they learn that beauty is not just skin deep.

In a sense, all cancer patients experience a sort of new birth. So often I hear the biblical phrase "passed from death to life" from them. They are often reduced to a state of vulnerability that they have not experienced since their birth. And for most, they become as bald as the day they *were first born*.

They must learn from those of us around them how they are perceived and valued in this world. If it is reasonable to tell Crumb Bunny how beautiful she is, to feed her righteous baby vanity, then the woman (or man) with cancer deserves no less. Whether stroking a shiny bald head or enjoying a thick new pelt, touch can make someone beautiful as well.

But how do we, the healthy, get beautified? We can choose the people whom we allow to influence us, seek those who can teach us life's most profound lessons. But there are risks. Jesus puts it this way, "Those who find their life will lose it, and those who lose their life for my sake will find it" (Matt. 10:39 NRSV).

If we wish to find out what life is all about, we had best not run from those people who threaten us. For me it was children with cancer. For you, there may be a different lovegiving, lifesaving embrace.

"Happy are they who bear their share of the world's pain," says Jesus. "In the long run they will know more happiness than those who avoid it."[1] It is more painful to stand at a "safe" distance than to be right there in the thick of it. The closer I am to these children, the more likely I am to be transformed by their radiance. By the time I retire, I expect to be a very beautiful woman.

13

The Color of Pain

God whispers to us in our pleasures . . . but shouts in
our pains: it is his megaphone to rouse a deaf world.

C. S. LEWIS

Dear Crumb Bunny,

Today is not one of your good days. Your poor mouth has
ulcers, and your little bum is so raw that you wail when you pee. I
hate to see you cry like that.

Your misery reminds me of all the painful tests I've had to
do on you over the last year. Your little mouth used to collapse into
a frown when you saw me come in the room. I think of all the ways
that I cope with your pain and what it is that keeps me from running from the room.

I face your pain by getting into my can-do medical mode,
dialing up the dose of morphine, looking ahead to when the sores
will heal. I know that just like the bone marrows and the spinal taps,
even this pain is just for a season. But do you?

Your mom comes right along when I do anything painful to
you. She and I chatter and think about how important the test is
rather than what it takes to do it. Years from now when you are

safe, we'll lose our need to chatter and laugh. But today, we must get you (and us) through.

You whimper in your sleep and I want to take your pain away forever and hurl it off this planet. What color for you is the color of pain?

———•

In our clinic, everything painful seems relative and each of us has our own way of coping. Most of our young friends are perfectly clear about the rank order of owies. There are finger-sticks and spinals. And then there's the dreaded bone marrow. Nobody likes a bone marrow.

Dip a brush in a pot of paint of as bold a shade of red as you can imagine. Hot tomato isn't a bad choice. Neither is crimson blaze. But blood-red. Ah, yes. Especially blood-red would make the point nicely.

Don't chintz in the sweep of your brush or the intensity of the shade if you want to be properly descriptive. Dracula blood-red. Start your sanguineous stroke where the hip bone's connected to the tail bone and then sweep over to the thigh bone, painting back and forth in radiating ruby rings.

This is pain that we're describing. When we're talking about the pain of a bone marrow, we should be suitably graphic if we would tell the truth. Sometimes the experience of pain can be expressed in words or colors. For severe pain, children see red.

Those of us whose job it is to treat the pain of children have the extra challenge of understanding pain in their own terms. We dare not think that a child's viewpoint is the same as our own.

Youngsters rarely think of medication as the solution for pain in a cause-and-effect manner. Their hope for pain relief comes on from more personal considerations. Psychological pain cannot be easily separated from the physical experience of a medical procedure.

There is an adage in pain-management circles that goes like this: "Pain is what the person with pain says it is." As a physician who must sometimes inflict pain on children, I am compelled to understand the length and breadth and height of pain from a child's point of view. I must posit myself with them if would help them with their distress.

Numerical scales are quantitative ways for clinicians to ask older children and adults to describe their pain. "On a scale of 1 to 10," we ask, "how would you rate your current pain?" On this scale, 1 is no pain and 10 is the worst pain you can imagine. If I were a four-year-old, all misery would be a 10. We call these kids our Sarah Heartburns, and we know more than a few little Sarahs.

Sarah comes to the treatment room tearfully and ver-rrrrrrrrrry slowly. Her thousand quasi-logical excuses en route might appeal to a very naïve parent, or pathetically young doctor, but we all lost our innocence long ago. Sarah knows that, so she holds back her trump card.

"Ah, Sarah!" I greet her, oozing with friendliness. "Hop right up here." She has gnawed her favorite security blanket threadbare so her mom makes a fast swap for number-two alternate from her Big Brown Bag. As our nurse's aide Esther lifts the child to the examining table, Sarah launches another small stall. I dare not let her catch me looking at my watch or I am dead meat.

I glove and paint Sarah's backside an iodine-rich brown. I am ready to start, a syringe of numbing Lidocaine loaded and lifted. Sarah murmurs, "I gotta pee."

I snicker and Sarah's tone becomes strident. "It's not funny. I *really* mean it." Too late, I try to abort a second-wave snicker rising in my throat, but she hears it and releases a warm stream of golden revenge.

Esther strips away the soaked surgical toweling and Sarah's undies. Mom pats her bag, locating the fresh change of clothing she always brings for the child. As I reglove to start over, Sarah warns, "Don't forget to say 1–2–3!" To control the controller is to control the pain.

A portion of Sarah's pain is the sadness with which her mother anticipates the procedure. Parents dread the possible test results as much as the instruments that invade their babies' tender flesh. We learned a valuable lesson about the actual physical pain of a bone marrow a few years ago.

One of our partners planned a research project that needed bone marrow from normal volunteers. A laboratory co-worker frequently volunteered. She was paid handsomely for her pain and always seemed prepared to donate again.

Our volunteer was able to control her own date with destiny, her certain knowledge that she did not have to think of bone-marrow aspirates as part of the rest of her life. She was not concerned how her bone marrow might look under the microscope, whether leukemia had relapsed. Her hope lay in her paycheck, not in the results. She was not at risk. She was sure and in control, and that is the way we prefer our lives to be.

In the course of my work, I frequently provide a second opinion for parents whose children are under treatment at other medical centers. In many cases, the recommendations of the first doctor were entirely appropriate and I wonder why the parents traveled so far to have their questions answered.

They have made the trip to rid themselves of pain. Sometimes I can relieve them by listening patiently to questions: Why was that scan done? My son was so frightened in that cold room by himself. Why was such a powerful medication given to so small a child? By honoring their need and right to know, I fill a yawning chasm that has been packed with their pain. I see the relief registering on their faces. But not all parents.

Some parents may seek to ease their pain by searching for someone who can eliminate all uncertainty. The comment of one mother with great mental anguish helped me see this more clearly.

Susan's daughter was first thought to have a highly lethal form of cancer. Had that diagnosis been correct, Tiffany would receive surgery, chemotherapy, and radiation according to a prescribed protocol. That treatment would be rough on the child but it most likely would have been curative.

Rather than cancer, Tiffany has a benign disease that may well go away on its own. Surgery, radiation, or chemotherapy can be held in reserve and are unlikely to be required. After several months of living with this benign but uncertain situation, Susan admitted that she was jealous of the parents in the same clinic whose children had cancer.

She (almost) wished that her daughter had certain malignancy rather than an uncertain future. It might even be easier to know that Tiffany will surely die than not to know how the story will end. Susan was not in control of her daughter's future, her own angst. She was seeing red. She was searching for someone who knew all the answers about her daughter's disease. Then, and only then, could she begin to relinquish control, learn the lessons of trust and uncertainty, to let go of her pain.

All worthwhile human relationships, whether with loving friend or respected physician, can only hint of a better way to trust. A wise man once said, "Trust in the LORD with all your heart, and do not rely on your own insight. In all your

170

ways acknowledge him, and he will make straight your paths" (Prov. 3:5–6 RSV).

As long as we keep seeking answers in ourselves or others to mollify our pain, we will fall back into the fear of uncertainty. There is a tension in trust, the knowledge that we must learn to trust and be trustworthy. Although a physician, I am only human, not much more certain than Susan. Parents and doctors alike, we must seek Someone worthy of our full trust, especially when the future is uncertain.

When I think about pain, I remember the heartbreak of a young mother and father listening to a diagnosis, prognosis, implications for their future. But this couple, Crumb Bunny's parents, moved past their pain and fought back. They armed themselves with a notebook, tape recorder, and telephone—parental tools of the medical martial arts. There were times that I was overwhelmed by their questions. But then I remembered that this was indeed war. I had hundreds of patients to care for and they had one surviving child. Let them fight their good fight. *For once, Di, be a simple foot-soldier instead of a general.*

Most parents who seek my advice are like these young parents and that is good. They master the art of advocacy for their children in ways that forge a healthy link with their doctors and fortify their other relationships. But on occasion, there is another sort of parent. Not fighters but flighters, they are running from even their necessary pain.

Cindy told me the case history without seeming to notice that her child was destroying my office. Her husband broke in often to correct her, all petty points. Mother and father talked at the same time, vied for my attention as their son, unregarded, vied for theirs. While the parents paralleled their monologues, Ricky used a red Magic Marker to spell out his pain on my white file cabinets, inscribing four-letter words that no four-year-old child should know how to spell.

There were only two points on which the parents seemed to converge. Rage ignited as Cindy talked about the first pediatrician. "Dr. High N. Mighty," she hissed. "He thinks he is God Almighty!"

Jack released his death-grip on his briefcase as he nodded in vigorous agreement with his wife for the first time. Their mutual hatred for this man, the tenuous glue that holds their fragile marriage together, is their single impetus to dialogue. Before the illness, it was the child himself who kept them together as a family.

With the threat to Ricky's life, they scramble to maintain their equilibrium. They'd scrambled thousands of miles that day to my office. If I failed to bellow their rage, I would be sending them away with less than they came for.

Jack opened his briefcase. His voice softened as he made a votive offering to me—a sheaf of publications about his son's disease, all from my pen. "You've written everything important that there is to say," he pleaded as he reached for his wife's hand. "You are the world's leading authority!"

I resisted the temptation to disburden their pain this way, quickly, easily. Somehow I had to assure them that their son would receive the best possible medical care without accepting oblation to my ego. They were asking me to play a more creditable imitation of God than the first doctor.

It is another one of those gray days when I must set out for Moriah to meet my newest Sarah and Abraham and Isaac. This new Isaac will survive—I've read that in his medical history—but will the family? If I do not fan the parents' fury, most likely they will find a third brittle point for accord. *Doctors always stick together*, they will say. *What could we have expected?* they will agree. For this and this alone, Jack will take his wife's hand. They will misunderstand my motive when I suggest that they examine their anger if they hope to get rid of the intolerable pain.

In *A Window to Heaven* I wrote of an operatic prologue that echoed a dying child's vision of angels. But it is not those angelic voices that I hear today. Rather, it is the satanic interruption from the same prologue that I recognize in this modern medical scene.

"Vainglorious dust! Overweening atoms!" complains Mephistopheles.[1] The master of evil is bored. Humankind is so debased that there is no one really worth tempting. But then he learns of Faust and Margereta, plots their undoing as man and woman, lovers, parents. Faust sells his soul for youth, Margereta murders their child.

Faust and Margereta, Abraham and Sarah, Cindy and Jack, Dr. Di and their doctor at home—Satan mocks us all. I detect his arrogant intrusion every time I face Mount Moriah. Two thousand years ago, on another pinnacle, that same sardonic laugh was heard and rebuffed:

> And the devil said to him, "To you I will give their glory and all this authority; for it has been given over to me, and I give it to anyone I please. If you, then, will worship me, it will all be yours." Jesus answered him, "It is written, 'Worship the Lord your God, and serve only him.'" (Luke 4:6–8 NRSV)

The first commandment remains simple, to have no other gods before God. Our task on Moriah is to learn what this means in our own families, in our own times, and in our own traditions. On Moriah we are alone with God.

Cindy and Jack are mere mortals. And they, like Abraham, are suffering mortal pain. Moriah's lesson seems perverse and cruel. I ache for the most important human beings in young Ricky's life. It would seem more merciful to extinguish their anguish, accept the offering, their glory, and all this authority.

But instead I must admit that I too am a pile of overweening atoms. I must point them away from me if I would offer real healing for their pain. I am reminded of words that were meant for all of us who hurt: "Come to me, all who labor and are heavy laden, and I will give you rest" (Matt. 11:28 RSV). These are not the words of a dusty demigod in white. They are an invitation from Christ.

Despite a hell on earth, Cindy and Jack are free to stop their flight. Abraham believed God and it was counted unto him as righteousness. Margereta and Faust repented and Mephistopheles was the loser. In the epilogue, it is the angelic chorus, the sweet sound of redemption, that fills our ears.

When Sarah's bone-marrow results are ready, I return to the treatment room with the good news that my little fighter is still in remission. The marrow was chock-full of robust, normal blood cells ready to fight infection, heal her bruises. Not one leukemic cell in sight.

Sarah listens to me, feigning disinterest, sniffing and smiling. Wordlessly, she grants her mother permission to launch preformed tears, heal her mother's pain. Mother dabs both pairs of eyes, echoes both sniff and smile.

I kiss Sarah on the forehead and push my luck a bit. "Now, tell me Sarah. Was that very bad?" I wait patiently, for to answer too quickly would not suit her mood or style.

"No, not really," she allows after an eternity-and-two-halves. Then she redeems me from my pain with a barely audible murmur, a sweet angelic whisper: "I wuv oo."

14

NIAP is Pain Spelled Backward

⟨≈❈≈⟩

As a mother comforts her child, so I will comfort you.
ISAIAH 66:13 (NIV)

Dear Crumb Bunny,

There's no need for a rooster in the Bone Marrow Unit as long as you are here. When you wake up, everybody rouses! You enjoy starting the day as the center of attention with a team of nurses hoping that you will smile and greet them. The other patients have to wait for their baths.

You've come to love these nurses so much that I can almost believe that you know that Mom and Dad need their rest.

"But it's the first time I'll be away from her overnight," Mom said as you were admitted.

"You've been on call in 'solo practice' for a year, Dr. Mom." I try my luck to convince her there are long-term benefits from short-term separation. "It's time for us to carry the beeper and you to get some rest."

Fortunately, Mom likes my metaphor.

You are so loved, and none of your lovers has ever paused to question your worthiness. Your pain is not so hard to banish. You *are apart from your mom and dad for a short season and then (in my fantasies) returned to their care until your wedding day.*

I wish it were so for all children.

The solution for much pain is not necessarily more medication. Before her bone-marrow transplantation, Crumb Bunny was hospitalized on the regular ward. Visits to that ward remind me that there are other forms of misery, with less hope than cancer, that can visit the young.

A six-week-old in a pram near the nurses' station is crying his heart out with a familiar howl. When I was an intern, we called them "baby junkies." Today they are known in our hospital vernacular as "jit babies," describing their irritable behavior as they withdraw from the narcotics their addict-mothers had abused.

The pain of withdrawal is handled with decreasing doses of narcotic and sedative but an important part of their therapy is never recorded on the chart as such. If the baby becomes too cranky, someone picks it up and holds it in her arms.

I take the infant from his tear-and-sweat-soaked sheet and the crying ceases as he is cradled snuggly, rocked gently. It's hard to rock and write, so my progress notes on charts on that ward have a peculiar jerky quality to the script. I am reminded of Luci Shaw's poem, *Mary's Song*:

Blue homespun and the bend of my breast
keep warm this small hot naked star
fallen to my arms. (Rest . . .
you who have had so far
to come.) Now nearness satisfies
the body of God sweetly.
Quiet he lies, whose vigor
hurled a universe. He sleeps
whose eyelids have not closed before.[1]

The baby's mother has returned to the streets to earn a living, abandoning him to our ward and the state. Some of these babies test positive for HIV as well, like the babe in my arms. He sleeps peacefully and I think of words attributed to Mary's hot naked star: *Whoever welcomes one such child in my name welcomes me*.

It is at times like this I think of my student days and my old chief. I wish he were still alive so that I could share these experiences with him. I recall one of the last times that I saw him before his death. On a day intended to honor him, some of his former students were invited to present scientific papers.

As I gave my medical paper, he beamed approvingly. I scanned the audience, looking for other familiar faces from the past. In the fourth row I spotted another now elderly, retired professor. He was scowling as he listened but I did not think he was disapproving. I was sure he was trying to fix me in time and place, this woman who works only with suffering children.

When science was sated, we adjourned to the faculty dining room for the festivities to continue. Science alone seemed inadequate praise for my old hero so I had composed a song. After lunch I took out my guitar and sang my *Ballad of the Silver Fox*. The chief was delighted. In the crowd I saw another older man, the one who considered pediatrics unsuitable for tender-hearted women. This time, a blaze of recognition transformed his features. He sought me out afterward. "Now I remember you," he said. "You always were a maverick."

The baby stirs in my arms. My paperwork is complete and I have no excuse to linger, so I rock a bit longer while I scan the horizon for another step-in parent to take my place. None is in view so I resume my rocking reverie.

The baby yawns expansively and tries his best to focus on me and the colorful squiggle pinned to my sweater that had brushed against his cheek. This brooch, a cheerful purple worm with blue stripes and a chartreuse bow tie, is my very own NIAP, gift of a teenager who contributed to its unique design.

NIAP is pronounced nape. NIAP is pain spelled backwards. As it says in the "owner's manual," every part of the NIAP is very important and has an important purpose. Like the curl on its tail (to help take away pain), the swirl on its body (to help take away boo-boos) and bright, bright colors—just plain nice to see.

The kids who designed it did so in the hope that its presence would assist everyone and anyone in their battle against all pain and hurt. I am one of the privileged few who have a NIAP to color-coordinate with almost any outfit I might wear. Color does not only describe the pain; it can spell out its relief as well.

Can I teach my own students to be the mavericks they were meant to be? An intern spots me with the baby and offers to take the next "shift." As my old chief encouraged me so many years ago to hasten Millie's healing by sharing myself, so I try to encourage the next generation of young doctors.

I kiss the soft sleeping head before passing him on to my maverick-in-training. The sweet perfume of baby shampoo lingers on my sweater as a reminder of how important human companionship is in the relief of pain.

15

Thwarting the Thief

⚜

The thief comes only to steal and kill and destroy; I [Jesus] have come that they might have life, and have it to the full.

JOHN 10:10 (NIV)

Dear Crumb Bunny,

My heart sank the day I first met you. The test results weren't back in yet but I knew what the diagnosis was. I've spent too many years stalking that thief. I know his MO all too well and so did your parents.

Your mother did everything possible to take care of herself and your brother-on-board during her first pregnancy. Except for the mild cold, everything had been perfect. But your brother was born critically ill, and they looked to your mother's history for the answer, wondering whether it was a virus. Mom and Dad laid your brother to rest after an autopsy, hearing that he was carried away by an overwhelming infection, a random piece of poor luck, not a repeatable event.

At least you were born healthy. But when the fevers began, the terror returned. You came to us, and your parents learned that the autopsy at the other hospital had missed the telltale cells. This was not random bad luck but a disease that kills one out of four of an affected babies' brothers and sisters. The thief was on your trail, seeking to rob you of your life, your parents of their only living child.

We temporized, shutting the thief out with chemotherapy and you revived to win all our hearts. But the thief knows the odds. The predator waits.

We are not satisfied with history repeating itself so we have hidden you away. That old robber cannot find you in our secret kingdom.

Each year I see a growing number of families who are poorly prepared for the long journey that lies ahead. There are too many opportunities for isolation available to the "me generation," and the solitary are sitting ducks for the thief.

On one of his old *Prairie Home Companion* radio shows, Garrison Keillor told of an experience at a folk concert. An artist thrilled his audience with a seemingly inspired rendition of "Amazing Grace." Keillor was touched by the performance and sought out the singer backstage. To his disappointment, the vocalist disclaimed that he actually believed any of the words he had just sung. The words had not come from his heart.

To express his disappointment, America's gentle contemporary humorist rewrote the lyrics of John Newton's famous old hymn. He composed an anthem suitable for today, an era that celebrates the self: *Amazing me, how sweet the sound.*

Keillor, enriched by grace, refused to let the thief rob him. While "amazing me" suggests introspection and isolation, amazing grace invites connection, reorients from I-I to I-thou and I-Thou.

A wealthy man was moving to our area. He visited various cancer centers to determine where his son would receive his further care. The boy still required chemotherapy and careful follow-up. The dad had already checked out each of our doctors. Now he was impressed with our new outpatient area.

This father seemed pleased until we reached the waiting area where a number of young African-American patients happened to be playing that day. The rich man's eyes narrowed and the pitch of his voice changed, "Of course, we will have to work everything around my son's schooling. We will want him to come at the end of the day so that he doesn't miss any classes. I can pay." His body language underlined his words. At the end of the day he hoped that these "other" children would be gone. He never came back.

This rich man let the thief rob him of a priceless treasure. His silver and gold could not buy the riches that we have to offer. There is no price tag on our greatest assets: ourselves and each other. And none of us, black or white, young or old, rich or poor, is less valuable in our family. You can't sneak in by a back door at night after potential "lepers" leave and still gain the best that we have to offer.

In the clinic where families mingle, friendships are solidified, and caring is extended to more than me and mine. There's an occasional solitary figure who slips in and out quickly without exchanging a word or glance with another, but that is the exception. No man, woman, child, or care-bear is an island here.

The mother of a boy with leukemia confided new insight about the communal aspect of the fight. Before her own child was hospitalized, she never knew another sick youngster. Where were they all—in some secret closet? Or was it she who had shut the door to these others and remained in narcissistic darkness until the door was blown open against her will?

This mother is not alone. Many parents of the newly diagnosed children ask if there is an epidemic of cancer in their neighborhood. They cannot believe that there always were this many young people with cancer. Until it affected them, they were blind to the extent of illness and suffering that others have already faced.

Sarah runs her hand over her own bald head as she clutches her security blanket shyly and approaches a teenager. "Do you have leukemia, too? You don't have any hair." Her nineteen-year-old new friend doesn't have leukemia, but he does have another form of cancer. Tom sits with Alff in his lap. He defies anyone to dare think that he is too old for stuffed stuff.

Tom sits next to his chauffeur-du-jour. This woman, wife of his pastor, clutches a teddy bear. She has an I-dare-you look on her face. By her side is the cane she uses to support herself during flare-ups of severely disabling arthritis. It could serve any shepherdess well, this beautifully carved and ornamented staff that expresses her defiance of the medical mundane. Alff's friend has a fine companion. Childlike but not childish, the pastor's wife is a one-woman crime-prevention unit. She would wonk the thief with her cane if he dared to approach young Tom.

When physicians concentrate only on the technical details of the physical illness, the robbery of grace is abetted. When nurses miss the interactions of body and soul, the loot fills the sack. When the family fails to move from amazing me to amazing grace, the thief emerges victor and moves on to the next victim. The joy of my work is to see how often the family is released from bondage and it is the thief who goes to jail.

16

Getting Airborne

I still get butterflies. They just fly in formation.
BRENDA LEE

Dear Crumb Bunny,

You come to your plastic window to greet me with your same sweet smile. You flap your arms by your sides making snow angels in the snow-pure laminar air. I mimic your motion to your delight. If you keep flapping, you'll rise out of your germ-free goldfish bowl!

You settle into your favorite sleeping posture, face turned away as if to shut out all but slumber, diaper-padded bottom raised in salute to the heavens. At this moment, you look very much like a baroque cherub to me. I reach my hand through the protective plastic glove to pat you. You shift slightly in your sleep, saying both "yes" and "no" to my embrace. For now, your dreams are your own.

Sweet dreams, Grandma's little angel.

Why is it that young children like my patients seem to soar in the heavenlies while adults such as I flop back down to earth regularly? Or even run. Pastor-author Browne Barr observes that geese fly much faster in formation than one by one.[1] It's tough flying by yourself. High-flying geese need fine-feathered companions. So do mere humans who face the valley of the shadow.

❧

In *A Window to Heaven*, I told the story of Naomi. Her dream surrounded her with the love of God in the moment that she knew that her baby would die of cancer. Naomi was so convinced that God's love would manifest itself in a plan for her life that she was content not to know if she would be given the gift of more babies.

It is now eight years since her firstborn died. God's plan has added two more healthy babies to their little family, and the youngest boy, Christian, is now three. At the dinner table he told Naomi, "An angel visited me last night. I liked him, so I invited him to stay the night and come to my birthday party."

It was Christmastime, a season whose symbolism richly recalls angel visitation. Intrigued, his mother inquired, "Did the angel stay the night?"

"No," answered the little one, then added, "He was a baby and he was very sick."

"What did the angel look like?" his astonished mother probed.

"Lots of lights, like a Christmas tree."

Naomi is a wise woman, one who knows when a three-year-old has closed a topic to further adult inquiry, so she allowed several months to pass before she again brought up Christian's angelic visitor. She asked him what the angel had told him. Christian became very quiet and said, "It's a secret."

I may be an adult, but I'm improving. In the company of these young children and their parents, I am losing my mistrust of things with wings.

What amazes me about my patients is how easily they understand what it means to keep the covenant, to be people of hope. Children who expect to live do not shrink away from those who will likely die. Their parents may find it a lot harder to maintain the closeness with less fortunate families, but they, too, try their best.

Parents of babies with Crumb Bunny's disease have banded together to help each other and help in research. The "FEL fighters" and "FEL angels" belong to the same family. Death does not have the power to separate these parents, to make them fear each other.

Matt had just started his treatment for Burkitt's lymphoma when he met Brian, who is now hospitalized for terminal care. Matt speaks lovingly of the lad, of his prayers for him. He is not afraid to maintain the attachment.

A few short months ago, Brian was hoping that the medicine would cure his cancer, but he did not shrink from visiting Sharon who was close to death. Three months after Sharon's death, her father visits Brian's mom. Brian, who knows that he is now dying, asks Sharon's dad if he has any messages for her in heaven.

The young artist whose paintings grace the jacket covers of my books is herself a recent addition to our hospital family. Not many months ago Korene came through a special form of surgery that removed her cancerous bone and, happily, saved her leg. Although her chances of survival are now 95 percent, she does not shy away from talking about those who did not survive. For Korene, hope means more than medicine and statistics, so she prays for Brian as well.

In the closing epilogue of *A Window to Heaven*, I acknowledged that I have unanswered questions for God about the death of children. To live with unanswered questions about the death of the very young requires grace to process hope. Baseball legend Dave Dravecky recently reminded me that grace is also needed for survivors. We talked about my young friend Korene, whose tumor is not unlike his that was removed by amputation, ending his baseball career. Dave thought about Korene and the other brave little players he personally knows. As he talked, his gaze drifted somewhere higher, another plane. He shared some important words of hope that have helped him get airborne:

> But we have this treasure in jars of clay to show that this all-surpassing power is from God and not from us. We are hard pressed on every side, but not crushed; perplexed, but not in despair; persecuted, but not abandoned; struck down, but not destroyed. We always carry around in our body the death of Jesus, so that the life of Jesus may also be revealed in our body. . . .
>
> Therefore we do not lose heart. Though outwardly we are wasting away, yet inwardly we are being renewed day by day. For our light and momentary troubles are achieving for us an eternal glory that far outweighs them all.
>
> So we fix our eyes not on what is seen, but on what is unseen. For what is seen is temporary, but what is unseen is eternal. (2 Cor. 4:7–10, 16–18 NIV)

Full of hope, my youngsters and the young-at-heart get airborne. Formation flying is natural for them, these lovers of life, my things with wings. And as hard-pressed, perplexed, crushed, persecuted, and struck down as I sometimes feel when I don't know all the answers, I will not lose heart. With them, I will fix my eyes on that which is eternal yet unseen.

Epilogue:

A Wedding Invitation

Gather the people. Sanctify the congregation; assemble the aged; gather the children, even infants at the breast. Let the bridegroom leave his room, and the bride her canopy.

JOEL 2:16 (NRSV)

Dear Crumb Bunny,

Today is a life-day that will always be remembered, a landmark medical and personal event. A stranger's marrow is flowing in your veins, introduced by an intravenous tube. Those foreign cells, looking for their new home, spell the difference between your death and your survival. How can anything lifesaving be truly foreign?

How fearfully and wonderfully made you are that these cells know where to go, the way to make both health and history!

You were born to be a history maker. Today will not be the last time. I plan to live long enough to be there on your wedding day. I can just see the headline:

BABY BONE-MARROW RECIPIENT BECOMES A BRIDE.

"Dr. Crumb Bunny was married today at Yale University's Dwight Chapel. The bride wore an ivory silk crêpe moire gown, edged with Victorian lace.

The wedding gown was hand-fashioned by her eighty-year-old doctor/grandma.

"The bride graduated with highest honors from Yale Medical School, receiving both M.D. and Ph.D. degrees.

"Dr. Crumb Bunny was awarded the Nobel Prize in Medicine for the identification and cloning of the gene responsible for familial erythrophagocytic lymphohistiocytosis, commonly known as FEL. She is the youngest Yale faculty member ever to receive this prestigious award.

"After a brief honeymoon in Florence, Italy, the couple will attend the International Congress for Gene Therapy for FEL in the same city. The bride will be the keynote speaker at the Congress."

I could fill your whole book with my dreams for you. Dreams are how princesses and grandmas get airborne.

Most of us chart our lives by mortal-but-sacred events. Births, baptisms, bar mitzvahs, graduations, weddings, death—all mark the familial, familiar rites of passage. These events are ancestral recipes, common but by no means mean. Suffused with spices that define their unique place in our families, they cut into our lives on purpose.

My favorite patient happenings are graduations and weddings. Especially weddings. For some patients, I have to wait what seems a lifetime for a meaningful spark of romance to ignite a good old-fashioned wedding. I suffer through the throes of young love with them and sometimes even assist with their dreams.

A two-year-old came to me from Nigeria, dying of widespread cancer. Chimma's mother would not take her back home without trying any treatment, despite my blunt statistical offering. The child's initial response to the chemotherapy I prescribed was prompt, but there was no reason to believe that she would not die from that tumor within a few brief years. This was no case for standard therapeutic recipes.

Six months later, Chimma was still doing well and I was invited to their cousin's wedding here in Connecticut. Her father sent a traditional Ibo dress and head-wrap for me to wear. At the reception, I was seated at the head table, my role as an honored guest-matriarch defined. I was to supervise the tossing of the bridal bouquet. In this regard, I am something of an expert. I probably hold the world's record for the most bouquets caught. I invited all the little girls to join in and, expert that I am, I knew exactly where the bouquet would land and so arranged my little patient's place in line. After giving the signal for the toss, I stood behind Chimma, guiding the bouquet into her hands. The other guests clucked their approval, sharing my hope that the child could live to be a bride. Her cousin's wedding day, the tossing of her bridal bouquet, were the first events that caused me to ask, "Why not?" Why couldn't Chimma live? Even with her zero statistical chance of survival, Chimma was entitled to hope.

Sometimes it takes symbolic days like wedding days to learn the right questions to ask, to design Books of Hope, and catch Hope Bouquets. In the paradoxical world in which I work, it is painfully easy to love children like Chimma and Crumb Bunny and all the others. You would love them, too, I wager, if you allowed yourself the risk of coming this close, as close as I am, and not worry whether they are guaranteed to survive.

Not long ago author Valerie Bell observed that it is not easy to love other people's children at all, even when they're healthy.[1] It doesn't seem to come naturally to us. I'd like to extend Valerie's thought further. It is not easy to love other people's adults. It isn't even easy to love your own adults!

Are you willing to stretch enough to love an adult or two that you currently despise, cherishing their company rather than fleeing from their presence? A covenant community wafts up to find other people's children and other people's adults and invite them along on the wing. It may not be easy, it may not even sound possible, but it is part of flying in formation as a people of hope.

Chimma caught that bridal bouquet twelve years ago. By all rights, she should be dead, but instead she's a lovely young teenager, smart as a fox. Her father faithfully sends me photos from Nigeria. Her youngest sister is named Diane.

In a few years I will watch my mail, waiting for a wedding invitation, wondering what the airfare is to Lagos that year. Meanwhile, I relish the letters, the photos, the news. All of it is good. In the Ibo tongue, Chimma means just that: "God is good."

This notion of wedding imagery to speak of the covenanting community is a biblical one. While I was in medical school, I became disenchanted with all such concepts, what I understood religious thought to be. Ironically, it was my experiences as a doctor at the bedsides of dying children that later led me to reconsider a Christian faith-profession. It was children who were dying who invited me to enter their covenant, to attend a marriage feast.

My youthful experience of Christianity left me so skeptical about most churches that I inclined toward a do-it-yourself, designer-religion. Organized religion seemed highly imperfect to me. I had my own cathedral, acres of virginal woods. I could read the Bible by myself, thank you, and commune with God in private. But it's hard to read that Book without looking for someone with whom its message can be shared. It's like attending a great performance alone and having no one to jab in the ribs when you get caught up in the ecstasy.

> Covenant commits more than the individual. God makes his covenant with Abraham, but through that covenant God brings a covenanted community into being that shoulders responsibility as a servant community to others. Otherwise, covenant deteriorates into the commitment of the loner, the physician as solitary gunslinger.[2]

Ironically, at the same time that I was wandering in the woods, I was telling parents of seriously ill children not to be lone gunslingers. I noticed that those parents in my practice who "made it" were those who linked themselves with people of kindred spirit, imperfect as those others might be. Finally, I heard the echo of my own words replayed. I recognized in its echo the discrepancy between my professional advice to parents and my own actions.

This lone gunslinger joined a local family of faith, imperfect as it may be, imperfect as I am. This faith-family has been my sounding board as I continue to seek to integrate my growing faith with my life's work. This is what covenant is all about: uniting with others, extending the invitation, preparing for the feast. It's no fun to dine alone. No bridal party invites only one guest.

The covenanted community is a ravishing bride, clothed in white fine linen, bright and pure. This is the image that John saw on the isle of Patmos, a gift-vision from a visitor with wings. "Blessed are those who are invited to the marriage supper of the Lamb," the angel said (Rev. 19:9, NRSV).

Because of the special children who have come into my life, I have set aside many of my presumptions. Things are not at all the way I had supposed. There is reason to hope. Life can defeat death, humor can stand in pathos' place. The weak and foolish lead, and I am often wise enough to follow.

Come, join me, then, dear friend. There's going to be a wedding. But first I must prepare, and so must you if you would come along. Leave your prejudices behind and take off your shoes, here on this holy ground. Don't even think about potential obstacles underfoot. Just lift up your eyes, fix and search for your goal.

You don't need answers to all your weighty questions to come along, only a passion for that which is unseen and eternal. And a heart full of hope. If you seem to lose your way en route to the feast, please don't despair. God knows your every need. He will send a child to lead you.

Hush, little Crumb Bunny. Grandma's here. The bone marrow infusion is now complete. Even though you don't notice, there's a change in you already.

You stand and clap to say hello. But, instead of saluting me with your backwards bye-bye, your tiny hand curves forward to tease me and to greet. Instead of your quaint little wave to yourself, for the first time your palm comes into view. The time has come, little angel, for you to share your secret.

You giggle and prance and show me something new. Finally, the reason for your preoccupation is revealed as you open your pudgy hand to greet me. For the first time I can see your big secret. It is God, unseen yet eternal, who is engraved on the palm of your hand. Come closer, little Sweetie. Come take my hand.

Love, Dr. Di

Afterword

Fourteen days after her bone-marrow transplantation, Crumb Bunny's blood counts started to indicate signs of new life coming from her bone marrow. In record time, her own bone marrow was making normal cells. The gracious gift of life had been accepted. She was now able to defend herself against infection and bleeding. It would not be long before the butterfly could be liberated from her sterile chrysalis.

The Tuesday after Easter, six weeks after her transplant, her mom entered the life island for the first time unmasked, ungloved, ungowned. It was my privilege to be there, on that holy ground.

"Can I kiss her?" she asked. It had been fifty-one days since this young mother was allowed to closely embrace her only living child. "I can actually kiss you!"

She clothed the baby in an Easter frock, bonnet, gloves, and slippers. Even her pacifier was color-coordinated. On her way out the door, Crumb Bunny paused briefly, admired herself in a mirror. She was plainly in awe.

Then the baby toddled out with her parents, not looking back.

Rebekah's Twins

1

Rebekah's Twins

⌘

When her time to give birth was at hand, there were
twins in her womb. The first came out red, his whole
body like a hairy mantle; so they named him Esau.
Afterward his brother came out, with his hand gripping
Esau's heel.

GENESIS 25: 24–25 (NRSV)

The welcoming ceremony was about to begin. It took
Becky longer than other mothers to move from the waiting
area to an examining room. First, she must traverse our clinic
gauntlet as all eyes converged on the peas from her proud pod.

At the nursing station, a spray of white dots on a dark
blue background wiggled onto the scales. "Are you really Ruth,
or are you Leah?" Nurse Peggy pleaded with the child, not
knowing if she was weighing the correct twin. Behind Peggy,
an inverse set of dots, blue on white, giggled. The nurse groped
for her eyeglasses, ceremoniously untangling them from her
necklace of keys and bandage scissors. Clearer eyesight did not
resolve her predicament, for she could not tell the girls apart.

Only one of the twins was my patient, but Peggy decided to weigh them both. She relished handing me a riddle with the chart: *Navy dots on white: 35 pounds; white dots on navy: 45 pounds.* Their mother always knew who was who, but not many other mortals shared Becky's certainty. Peggy counted herself among the ranks of mere mortals. In most ways, Ruth and Leah were indistinguishable, from the teasing gray eyes to the missing front teeth. But there was a consequential disparity: Only Ruth had leukemia.

It was easier to tell the girls apart when Ruth was going through the intensive part of her chemotherapy. Leah was the one with curly blonde hair. Ruth was the one who said, "If you're nice, I'll let you stroke my silky bald head." But now her hair is fully regrown. Now you have to wait for the dreaded pulse of prednisone for the scales and Ruth's chipmunk cheeks to tip off the difference. Doctors and nurses from other specialty clinics paused in their own activities to join the parade, as if they would miss a mitzvah if they failed to greet Ruth and Leah. I smiled myself at the mystery—that outsiders yearn to linger and comment. Unmitigated strangers feel entitled—nay, obligated—to gape at Mother Nature's miracle mirror. I chided myself for joining in the voyeurism. *They are two individuals*, I told myself, *not two halves of one child.* Each needs to be respected for who she is. But I missed Leah if she did not come with her sister, for there seemed to be something lost.

Joey's mother was in the clinic that particular day. Her own child, immersed in a Nintendo game, ignored her. "Who's Ruth, and who's Leah?" she queried. The girls sighed, refusing to enlighten their inquisitor. As long as there will be twins, there will be inquisitors. It was anyone's guess that day which was Leah and which was Ruth. When I walked in the room, I shook my head incredulously at the vision of frilly white panties before me. Ruth had swooped down to recover a fallen toy from the floor, offering the entire staff a ruffled peep show, encouraging my thoughts to wander home.

A painting hangs over my fireplace at home. In a lovely garden scene, watercolors shimmer in the freshness of summer sunshine. Hollyhocks sway in a mild breeze as if they are there to set the rhythm for two figures we see at work. Only the blossoms behold the children's faces. The artist leaves us to surmise what the snapdragons surely know. Little girls about the age of Ruth and Leah stand with their backs toward us. Twin sisters, they are pinning laundry onto a backyard clothesline. We see only silky pale-blonde hair, starched candy-stripe dresses, and white multi-layered frills peeking out from beneath. In the painting, one child bends from the waist, picking dolls' clothes out of a basket.

For many years this picture was a source of family controversy. It still is. Since you cannot see the faces, even those who allege inerrant discernment cannot say for certain which twin it is. My sister and I each contend that it is the other whose ruffled derriere salutes the spectator.

The watercolor was based on one of many prize-winning photos that my father took of us in our childhood. A grandaunt in Chicago was the artist who transformed our urban driveway into a country garden with the aroma of roses and Rinso White.

The painting hung prominently in my parents' home when we were children. Today it hangs in mine. As a child, I hated for people to see it. There was the inevitable question that followed, asked only of The Twins. Which one of us was bent over? Guests in our home never seemed to ask our parents. The dreaded question was always directed to The Twins.

When we were growing up, my sister and I weren't just Di and Marge. To the rest of the world, we were the Komp twins. Or, more simply, just The Twins.

Becky greeted the other mothers in the chemo room. Once, she—and these other women—had had an identity apart from their children. But that seemed a different lifetime, long since discarded. Mornings like these, she huddled with other waiting women and the occasional father who brought his child. When it was "just girls" in the room, intimacies were shared as if they had known each other for their entire lives.

Becky would have preferred to marry right after college, but her parents prevailed on her to wait and take her time. She taught social studies for a few years at a junior-high school in the Bronx until she met a fellow teacher named Manny. He shared her dreams for a large family. After their honeymoon, she composed an undated letter of resignation, ready to offer it to the principal when she became pregnant. Weekends, she and Manny drove north of the city in search of a house large enough for all of her dreams.

Many of her Hunter College chums talked of waiting till they were firmly established in their careers before they began their families. Not Becky. Like her Grandma Selma, Becky imagined presiding over a houseful of children. Each year her hopes for a family dwindled and her teaching contract was renewed. Eventually, she stopped going to her college reunions. Even her friends who planned to wait were now immersed in parenting. Becky was pained by the exclusivity of their baby talk. Everywhere, there seemed to be a reminder of what she did not have. Even away from home. On the beach where they vacationed, she always noted the babies. Her husband was at a loss about how to relieve his wife of her emptiness.

Eventually, Becky quit the school in the Bronx, and they moved to a small house in Cos Cob. She was about to sign a teaching contract for a school in Connecticut when she became pregnant. No longer barren, Becky gladly retired from the work world. She reinvested in her original dreams and commingled her own identity with that of her impending issue. Rebekah was to be the mother of twins!

Near the end of her pregnancy, Becky could hardly move. At night she lay in bed like a massive lump as she and Manny watched the late-night belly-war. Her husband tenderly stroked the spot where the last blow seemed to surface. "Hey, you guys in there!" he would call into her inverted navel. "It's time to go to sleep. You can pick up the battle tomorrow." Becky wondered what they thought they were competing for.

Mother and father were both exhausted from the nightly baby fistfights. When the twins weren't punching each other out, they were tap dancing on Becky's bladder. She was secretly relieved when they were born ahead of their due date.

Leah came easily and was the first to be born. But Ruth was a breech baby, bum first. Out of it all were born their new, unique identities. "Baby Girl A" and "Baby Girl B" metamorphosized into The Twins. And Rebekah became known as The Mother of The Twins.

She savored her new role in life. Becky felt unique, respected, admired, novel, proud. Her tiny daughters stared across her body when they nursed, their infant eyes trying so hard to converge on that other self. But when they cried, Becky imagined that they picked up their argument where they had left off *in utero*. Is it possible that two babies can sound louder than one plus one?

Manny nicknamed his wife "The Great Equalizer," as she spent all her energy trying to make sure neither child had more than the other. For the first three years her happiness was interrupted only by childish squabbles. It seemed that the harder she struggled to keep them equal, the more the children struggled to pull apart. Then, one day, Leah hit Ruth, and a nosebleed began that would not stop.

That was how the leukemia started. Both girls were there when I came to the Emergency Room late that night. Ruth lay like a silent slab of stone on the hospital gurney. Leah was screeching and scratching at her mother's face. Becky went with me to the treatment room when I did the test that confirmed their pediatrician's suspicion and her own worst fear. Ruth was so weak that she did not even struggle.

Leah remained with Manny, howling the whole time. "I want my mommy," she cried and was clearly heard through the closed door. This brutalized Becky more than any pain that Ruth might receive at my hand. She felt torn in half. Over the weeks to come, I noticed something unusual in their relationship. I'd dealt with dozens of pairs of twins as patients, but this was the first time I ever felt a tension between the two. Some cling closer to their twin than they do to their parents, unable to tolerate the briefest separation. But Ruth and Leah wanted to separate from each other, each tugging Becky in her own direction. In turn, Becky tried to pull and push them back toward each other. Their mother invested much of her energy into this grand-scale balancing act.

Once leukemia came into their home, Becky interpreted a simple sibling row as a risk to Ruth's life. When the inevitable squabble erupted, Leah was always questioned and usually blamed. Ruth relished her position as victim, first in her mother's concerns. As time passed, Leah became more sullen.

Her favorite line was, "It's not fair!" Frequently, it wasn't. Most of the major brouhahas occurred in private. For the masses, The Mother held court and The Twins held their tongues. They knew their mother's expectations. Both children came for every clinic visit. I suspected that Leah prized the attention more than Ruth. She certainly had less to suffer for the encounter. Only once did we take blood from her. Usually, she was there to entertain and be entertained.

Ruth's health returned quickly, and her visits became reasonably routine. Her treatment plan was for three years of chemotherapy, daily pills, and less frequent shots. We had every reason to expect that she would be one of the fortunate children with acute lymphoblastic leukemia to survive.

Becky never shared my optimism. From the very beginning, she wanted to plan for a relapse. It was in this context that we drew blood from Leah, confirming her eligibility as a bone-marrow donor. Becky congratulated Leah. If Ruth relapsed, she would save her sister's life.

$\sim\!\!\sim$

From time to time, Becky and I sat down together for tea and twin-talk. "Are you and your sister close?" she asked. Her question caught me off-guard. Most twin-mothers simply ask me if we still look alike.

"No, not really," I had to admit. "Sometimes I think that we're closer now than when we were younger. Perhaps because we live at a distance, the miles give us more room to breathe."

These conversations tended to be brief, but Becky never let me drop the subject without asking about my mother, what it was like for her to be The Mother of The Twins. My mother was an only child who wanted more than anything else to have a large family. She had great difficulty conceiving, and then only once did she become pregnant. In a way, God answered her heart's desire with the twin pregnancy. She didn't want to mother an only child. "But what was it *really* like for her?" Becky pushed. "Did she ever tell you?" Becky was asking not the mother but the daughter. Can a child ever truly speak for the mother, cut the cord, step back, and take a clearer, cleaner look?

My mother (who died more than twenty years ago) loved to talk about being a mother. While growing up, I heard her recite the details of her pregnancy many times over. These were the stories that I remember, the apotheosis of her blossoming double burden. Many of her stories began, "When you and your sister . . ." My mother loved being The Mother of The Twins.

At our hospital all our little patients have rituals. Ruth and Leah were no different. When I entered the examining room, I was supposed to guess if the correct twin was sitting on the table. I never erred. I said that it was my powers as a twin that guided me. It was actually a slightly coarser turn to Ruth's curls when they regrew after chemotherapy. It took a clinically practiced eye to mark the difference. None of the other doctors shared my discernment. The Twins believed in the secret power of another twin. Sometimes I played along, dutifully examining Leah. I frowned when I palpated her belly, *hummmmmmmmmmmmed* for the longest time when I auscultated her chest. "Okay, Ruth," I said, "there's something else I need to check. I know you're in a hurry today, so I'm not going to send you back to the lab. Just let me draw your blood right here and now."

Leah shrieked, Ruth squealed, and Becky dutifully reported that I had the wrong twin. Simultaneously both girls said, "Or did you know all along?" I simply grinned my omniscient twin-grin.

The twins were settled in together in the chemo room on a lounge chair watching *The Little Mermaid* when I walked with Becky to our kitchenette.

"What was it like for you growing up?" she asked, looking into her teacup. Was she a psychotherapist or the mother of one of my patients? I grubbed through old memories, unearthed something of that which she sought. On the Christmas Eve that came to mind, snow was falling.

We lived in an old brownstone in Brooklyn then, not far from where Becky herself grew up. Many of the rooms railroad-carred into each other by a door through to the next room. I can't remember which room our private elves operated from. Whichever, on Christmas Eve, that room was off-limits to The Twins.

On childhood's most wondrous night of the year, I snuggled in bed listening for Christmas noises. I could hear Mom and Grandma chatting softly, accompanied by the whirring obbligato of an ancient Singer sewing machine. Their muffled voices moved in chanting waves over the surge and ebb of the next seam.

They would stay up all night, I imagined, sewing for us. Christmas morning, the world's best-dressed twin dolls sat under the tree, waiting for adoption. Our beaming elves stood by, waiting to see our faces when we saw the dresses they had made for us as well. After breakfast, they signaled Dad to put down the Brooklyn Eagle and get his camera gear. Mom and her mom were most content when they were working together. Grandma was an eighteen-year-old war widow when her only child was born. It was as if they had grown up together, two sisters. My grandmother had lived with us for as long as I could remember.

"Mom and Grandma were closer than Marge and I ever were," I told Becky. "I think closer than we will ever be." My grandmother outlived breast cancer, even metastases. Saddest for her, she even outlived her daughter. That was never her intention. I never heard her grieve. I simply felt her pain. Two years after my mother's death, I saw her smile return briefly when she held my sister's firstborn baby in her arms. A few days later, she didn't wake up.

Becky dug some more, calling me abruptly back to the present. "Do you remember what your mother said when you and your sister fought?"

It isn't words that I remember. It was a profound sadness that Becky had dredged up. Mom didn't get angry very often. When we fought, I remember my mother's looking as if she had been mortally wounded.

When Ruth and Leah started school, I was firm with Becky. Ruth was doing well, and her visits were fairly routine, but both children missed a day of school when the child with leukemia needed to be seen.

Becky and I skirmished over this school issue. There was a big chicken-pox epidemic one year, and she wanted to keep both girls out of school the entire year. I declined to sign a document for home schooling for the healthy child. I recommended that Leah be sent to school even if she got ahead of Ruth in her studies.

Unfortunately for her, it was Leah who developed chicken pox first. She was persona non grata in Cos Cob that week. Becky sent her into exile with Manny at an aunt's house on Long Island so that she would not further expose Ruth.

Their mother acidly pointed out that Leah had been exposed on the school bus on one of the days she went to school and Ruth went alone to the clinic.

It was actually better for Ruth that we knew in advance exactly when she had been exposed. If both children had been exposed on the school bus without our knowledge, it could have been a lot worse. We were able to give Ruth a special gamma globulin in time. This medical clarification did not win points with Becky. There are times when logic goes unappreciated.

Poor Leah had a high fever and full-blown case, but Becky only visited her by phone. She was afraid that she would bring the virus home on her hands even if she wore surgical gloves when she touched her daughter. At home, she examined Ruth daily, looking for evidence of the scourge she feared. Three weeks after Leah, Ruth broke out with a grand total of two pocks. The gamma globulin had prevented a serious case. The rest was neutralized by an antiviral medicine. Ruth never even itched, but Leah returned from exile scabbed, scarred, and surly.

There were little warning signals about Leah's wretchedness. The Twins were squabbling over the same toy one day when I walked into the examining room.

"I hate you!" Leah spat at her sister. "I wish you were dead."

I proposed a sibling support group for Leah, but Becky overruled my suggestion. She wanted a group where both children could be together. I wondered whether Leah would feel free in such a setting, or if the two would simply perform as The Twins. No matter how much my sister and I battled in private, we pulled together when we felt threatened. It was the two of us against the world. In public, we were always The Twins.

Ruth remained in remission, and her visits became less frequent. Then, unexpectedly, five years after she was first diagnosed, she relapsed. We set the plans in motion for a bone-marrow transplantation. Leah, her twin, was a perfect match.

The donation itself is done under general anesthesia because of the pain and length of the procedure. Although parents must give the legal consent, a child who is old enough to understand what it all means is invited to give her own assent. Thus, the team talked to Leah about what lay ahead.

None of us was prepared for what followed. Leah was terrified that she would go to sleep and not wake up. It didn't matter to her that that had never happened to any donor we knew. Social workers and child psychiatrists, determined to be her friends and advocates, all talked to Leah, but she remained firm and fearful.

It did not help in the least that I had shepherded countless families through difficult choices over the years. As many families of twins as I had dealt with, this was a novel dilemma. Becky was beside herself with anger. She could not bear to be in Leah's presence.

"She's a child," she thundered. "She doesn't know what she wants or doesn't want. Her sister could die while she enjoys a temper tantrum. We're their parents. Why can't we make that decision alone?"

I tried in vain to explain how important Leah's feelings were in all of this. Leah remained firm in her refusal. I imagined what it would have meant if it were my sister who might die. Sometimes we made casual jokes like, *I'll lend you a kidney if you lend me your bone marrow.* But that was the jesting of adult twins. I tried to remember what it might have been like when we were eight years old ourselves. I cannot believe that one of us would have refused.

Once my sister nearly died. In our senior year in college, an inexperienced driver panicked in the fog. He let go of the steering wheel to shield his own face and hit a carful of student teachers head-on. My sister was one of them, riding in the suicide seat that day. She went through the windshield.

It was a Thanksgiving weekend when I caught a ride to far-off Indiana. We had agreed on separate colleges, almost a thousand miles apart. I remember seeing her bandaged face and newly rewired jaw. I can visualize the hospital chapel where I wept and prayed (I've never told her that). If worse had come to worst, I would never have refused to save her life. I may not have found the words, but I surely would have found the deed.

Sibling rivalry, parental favoritism—these are common parts of family life but not ordinarily matters of life and death. Usually, the matter of bone-marrow donation is a voluntary act of a consenting adult, but this case involved two minor children. No matter what drama ruled their private lives, the medical staff had to ensure that both children's needs and rights were protected.

I tried talking to Leah without pressuring her, twin to twin. Her resentment was deep-seated. Leah was certain that Becky would sacrifice her for Ruth. Ever since her sister became ill, the child was aware of her mother's expectations. She recited them like a venomous litany. Leah believed that her mother loved her sister more. Leah interpreted Becky's efforts to restore parity as gross inequity.

My heart went out to the child we could not seem to help. The first steps toward the transplant needed to be set in motion long before we knew if it would ever actually happen. Unknown to Becky, this time of preparation turned into years in which Leah felt robbed of her birthright.

But as things turned out, Leah experienced all the pressure of deciding without ever having to donate. Ruth wasn't responding to chemotherapy and remained in the hospital, suffering one grim infection after another. Leukemic cells continued to grow through the most effective chemotherapy we knew. She wasn't going to survive long enough to receive anyone's marrow.

We reached the point where the institution of hospice home care would have been an appropriate choice. This was a bitter burden for Becky. She counted on the transplant and refused to consider withdrawing intensive chemotherapy. I lamented for the child who was confined to a hospital bed rather than liberated for her final days at home. I asked Becky if Leah wanted to come to visit her sister. I hadn't seen her in more than a week. Their mother's eyes filled with tears.

"It's not fair," she mourned. "All I ever wanted was to be the mother of twins. If Ruth dies . . ." She folded into my arms as we both struggled for words.

"You will always be The Mother of The Twins," I told her. "If they had both survived, someday they would have moved out of your home. Whether it be to college, or to live with husbands, the day would have come when all you would have at home is your memories. Even if the time you've had was shorter than you had expected, no one can take that away from you."

Becky moved to the windowsill, looking out as she spoke. "I know this sounds silly," she continued, "but I won't be special anymore. As the mother of twins I felt unique." She turned back toward me, gasping, "Save my daughter!" Her gasp dissolved into a sob.

"I wish to God I could save her, Becky." *How many times have I said those words?* "But whether Ruth lives or dies, you are unique. Each of us is. Even Ruth and even Leah. It's a paradox."

"Is that what this twin business is?" she asked. "A paradox?"

Yes, perhaps, I thought. *Paradox is the only word that seems to make sense.*

᠁

On Friday evening, Ruth lay dying. "The time has come to ask her what will make her happiest," I told Becky. The child asked to see her sister, and Manny brought her there.

The children didn't speak to each other. Leah simply crawled into the bed with Ruth, each folded toward the other. It was as if they had womb-work left to do. I never heard them speak a word.

Manny and Becky stood there on that Shabbat evening, blessing Ruth and Leah. *May God bless you and protect you. May God look your way and be gracious to you. May God favor you and bring you peace.* Manny held his wife as the twins held each other, until Ruth died. Then Becky climbed into the bed and held both her daughters, one cradled in each arm. And their father embraced them all.

᠁

It was two years later that I heard a timid tap on my office door and turned to find Leah. Our sibling support group was meeting that afternoon. She had asked Becky if she could come.

"What a wonderful surprise!" I said, opening the door wide. Becky signaled that she was going to call on our social worker while her daughter visited with me. Leah sat down in a chair, pulled it close to mine.

She looked around my office—a child-friendly place. I'm very proud of the love-gifts that fill my work space. There are children's paintings on every wall, each with a wonderful story. It was something on my desk that caught her attention, caused her to stand, reach, bring it closer. It was a silver-framed photo of two young boys. "Are they your sons or your sister's?" she asked. Most people would have assumed that the boys were mine.

"That's Mitch and Scotty. They're my sister's boys."

She looked around my desk for another picture and did not find what she sought. "Is your sister still alive?" she asked, a ten-year-old child who took nothing for granted! I reassured her that Marge was alive and well.

"Do you and your sister still look like twins?" she wondered, relaxing back into the chair, still examining the photo of my nephews.

"No, not really," I admitted. "I guess we could if we didn't fool around with our hair color and our weight didn't go up and down at different times. But we have a lot of the same mannerisms. Mitch and Scotty notice that.

"When they were younger," I remembered, "the boys used to shake their heads and say, 'It's not just that you look like Mommy!'" Leah giggled, realizing that the twin business can go on for a lifetime. And beyond.

"Are you and your sister close?" She was Becky's daughter!

"I don't think you could really say that, Leah. It wasn't always fun for us to be twins. In fact, there were times when it was downright hard." She nodded wisely. She seemed so young to be struggling with thoughts that were only feelings for me at her age. She picked up another picture off my desk.

"Is that your mother?" She had located the other Mother of The Twins. "Did she make you dress alike?" she asked. You'd better believe it!

My sister and I finally rebelled in high school, one leaving the house earlier in the morning so that Mom wouldn't see that we weren't dressed alike. Strange—now we buy each other identical dresses. "It was hard for me to be a twin," Leah said. "Now it's even harder not to be. But I think it's harder for Mommy than for me." The child rose from her chair, walked to the window. "Sometimes I wonder whether Mommy can love just me," she said sadly.

"I'm sure she can, Leah," I offered. "But for your mom, being The Mother of The Twins was what made her feel special. In a way, you and your mom face the same struggle. When you're a twin, you're unique because there aren't many other twins around." I was thinking out loud again. "But then you're not unique, because there's another one just like you. And your mom has the same struggle."

I didn't know if the child would understand me, but I needed to work it out for myself. She turned from the window and laced her arms around my neck from behind. I was grateful for the small, warm hands, the soft reminder that I was not alone.

"It's sad," I told her, "but nobody much treats moms as special." It was not just Becky's face that filled a mother-sized space in my heart but the portrait of every woman who has come back to this office after a child's death, drawn back to a place where she was treated with respect, blessed for simply being who she was. A mother. *Honor thy mother that thy days may be long in the land*. Perhaps, if we truly honored mothers, blessed them, the Beckys of this world would not feel that something more than their child had died.

I rose from my chair and took the child in my arms, winding down my monologue on twinnery. Leah was no longer the three-year-old I first met. Nor the eight-year-old I knew when her sister died. She was almost a young woman. Someday she, too, may be a mother. I hope so.

"Leah, you are one of the most special women I've ever met in my entire life." I was telling the truth. "In some way, Ruth will always be part of you. It's almost as if I can hear her saying, *Blessings on you, my sister. I will always be with you, but I want you to be free to be you. Peace, my dear sister.*"

She lingered for a while in my arms. Then, she was ready to go. With a final glance at a painting on my office wall, she added, "The next time I come, I'll bring you one of my drawings." With that benediction, she withdrew from my office.

I walked to the office door and saw her farther on down the hall. She was standing arm in arm with Becky, talking to one of the nurses.

"Did I ever tell you how special my mom is?" the child asked the nurse, blessing her mother. "My mom is absolutely one of a kind."

Becky drew her daughter to her as they walked out together.

2

Mary Meets Martha

*As they went on their way, Jesus came to a certain vil-
lage, where a woman named Martha welcomed him
into her home. She had a sister named Mary, who sat
at the Lord's feet and listened to what he was saying.*
LUKE 10:38–39 (NRSV)

I never worried about my clinic schedule's starting on
time if Teddy Campbell's name was on the list. His mother
always asked for the earliest possible appointment of the day.
Long before the receptionist arrived, she and Teddy were there
in the waiting area.

Martha wanted to be the first in line when the lab
opened and the blood-drawing team looked for the first
patient. Just fifteen minutes later, all the other patients would
start drifting into the lab. It would be an hour before the full
results for any of them would be known.

When I entered the examining room, Martha greeted
me with Teddy's completed blood report. The day's results
were already recorded in a notebook she had kept ever since
Teddy's treatment began. With each new rotation of medical

students, I must teach them how to interpret those numbers. Martha learned to make the calculations the day her son's treatment began. That's the way I like my days to begin.

At first, our techs refused to give reports to a parent for fear that we doctors would disapprove. But it wasn't worth the effort to argue with Martha week after week. For her peace of mind, she must have all the blood counts before she could leave for home. For her, there was worth in these values, consolation that could be quantified. And I had to admit that her exigency sped up my work day. When I couldn't find Teddy's medical chart, I would beg a peek at Martha's flow sheets.

When Mary Bonito finally gets to the clinic with Sarah, the nurses are always glancing at the clock, sharing knowing looks. There is no way they can start up the baby's chemotherapy and still get to lunch themselves. Every week Mary asks for the latest possible appointment, but she never seems to make even that on time. A nurse comes to the doctor's conference room and begs me to talk to Mary again about punctuality.

Mary's stories don't vary much. She waited with her oldest son for the school bus, which, as usual, was late. Then, at the baby-sitter's house, there was a tearful farewell scene with her preschooler. Both boys have been afraid to leave Mary's side since Sarah was first admitted to the hospital. Mary wants them to know that she will always be there for them as well as their little sister.

The doctors for the next speciality clinic come drifting into the conference room, meaning to displace me as their own clinic is about to begin. "Why do your clinics always seem to run so late?" they grouch.

Nine-year-old Teddy and nine-month-old Sarah have the same disease. They came to us on the very same day, both suffering from a highly lethal form of neuroblastoma. Even their chemotherapy was the same. But their mothers were as different as midnight and daybreak.

Martha keeps in regular touch with parents at three other major treatment centers, comparing notes on treatment protocols. She shares with them what she learns from Teddy's doctors about the newest research. She asks other mothers about doses of the drugs their children receive so that she can enter it into her records.

The only mothers that Mary seeks out are those in the chemo room and the parents' support group. The medical details hold no import for her. Mostly, she concerns herself with how the other moms are doing, whether their children are happy.

Sarah and Teddy became ill at the same time and came to the same hospital. There the similarity seems to end, because Mary and Martha are as different as a fast and a feast.

When Teddy was born, Martha and Roger were ready. The young couple waited until they were financially secure before they started their family. They owned their first home, fully furnished. Everything—even Teddy—had been planned.

Roger liked his life in order, and Martha provided that order single-handedly. The other men in the office joked that their wives were more familiar with Montel Williams than Mr. Clean. Roger's buddies grumbled about the wages paid the latest maid. Martha's husband would never have to pay for a house-keeper. There was no one here on earth who could meet his wife's expectations. He had married a Lysol Lil who hoovered the floors twice a day. Nothing in their home was out of place.

The birth of their second child three years after Teddy brought a brief moment of disorder into the otherwise perfectly run household. Martha recovered quickly, brought all again into order. There was further slight discord when her sister came to help with Teddy, while Martha cared for the new baby.

The visit was shorter than originally scheduled. Martha's sister, Janet, liked to sit down after dinner. She would relax rather than immediately jump up to do the dishes. But Martha liked to load the dishwasher even before dessert was served. Roger had no grievance with sploshing while he was eating. It was dinner music for an antiseptic household.

The sisters' concepts of housekeeping didn't mesh. Janet felt she was there to assist, not to be converted. She left after three days, but no one really missed her for Martha could manage by herself.

Mary and Pete didn't plan her pregnancies. Their children just happily happened. Sarah was their third in six years, the baby of the family and the only girl. By the time little Sarah arrived, cheery mayhem had ruled their home for so long that Pete could not remember the last time he had seen an uncluttered house.

When guests appeared at the door, major obstacles were removed from the living-room floor. Someone briefly checked under sofa pillows to ensure that the dog hadn't buried any of his biscuits there. Humphrey waxed indignant if a visitor sat too close to his treasure trove. Naive guests sometimes found themselves jowl-to-jowl with a pouting basset hound.

Pete and the animal came to the marriage together, two happy ex-bachelors. With two little ones in Pampers, Humphrey had his employments. Nose a-twitch, he prowled after rug-rats, sniffing and snitching, fixing on terminal targets until change was transacted. Then Humphrey trailed all the way to the diaper pail (chained shut to keep him out).

With each successive pregnancy, Pete seemed to pick up momentum when other men might have found the novelty was wearing off. By the time Mary gave birth to Sarah, he and the other ex-bachelor had taken over the household. Pete placed the dirty dishes in the refrigerator, reasoning that it would control microbial overgrowth until he was ready to wash them. A handheld Dust Buster sufficed to suck the crumbs off the kitchen floor. Humphrey's tongue followed Pete's hand, slicking the linoleum to a high polish.

Mary's merry men curled up after supper to watch football on the tube. Humphrey's rump and Pete's lap pillowed the children's heads. By halftime, all four were snoring in concert. Mary's mother came a few days later, rescuing the family from the Pizza Taxi.

Pete never seemed to tire of the wonder of a newborn's entry into life. When the new mom came home from the hospital, he brought her breakfast in bed. He raced home from work in the middle of the day to watch his wife breast-feed his new daughter. He overstayed his lunch hour many a day, for Pete was a happy man.

For Teddy, the illness began with an aching in his bones that kept him awake at night. Martha rocked him in her arms and sang to him. Nothing she could do seemed to help. The first pediatrician called it "growing pains." There was nothing to prescribe other than Tylenol. Martha had already tried that and begged for something stronger. The child was not a complainer. It was not like him to cry out in the night.

She changed doctors. The second pediatrician suggested arthritis as the diagnosis. Martha became frantic as her son became sicker and she received no answer that helped.

Teddy lost three pounds the last week before he came to us. The child was unable to eat by day. He cried in his sleep at night. Roger became irritable from the loss of sleep. He was easy to get along with when his life was in order, but he had low tolerance for disorder. Their entire married life, Martha had always been able to keep perfect order for them both. This was the first time that everything wasn't in her control.

Annabelle stopped by one day for coffee and found Martha hysterical in her own kitchen, repeating to herself, "Stay calm. Keep in control. Don't lose it." Her neighbor touched her hand, but Martha pulled away abruptly.

"No, I'm okay. I just didn't get very much sleep last night. Teddy seems so sick, and none of the doctors seems to know what's going on." It was then that Teddy cried out in such agony that Martha flew up the stairs, sobbing.

"I'm taking you to the Emergency Room, right now," Annabelle said and headed next door to get her car keys. It was there that Martha first heard the terrible word.

The pediatrician who examined Teddy took her to Radiology so that she could see the X-ray film for herself. On a back-lit view box, she saw white shadows on black. They meant nothing to her.

"Do you see, here and here?" he asked, pointing to what seemed like thigh bones. It was Teddy's legs they had photographed. "This should be all white, but the bones look moth-eaten, both legs."

He flipped a switch, lighting the next panel. More shadows, this time of the boy's body. "And here, on the belly films. This white area shouldn't be there. This is what's causing his pain. We think it's a tumor, a form of cancer."

Cancer! It was then that Martha knew that if Teddy would survive—if she would survive—she must get control of herself. Of all times in her life, this was the most important time that she be in control.

❧

She was bathing the baby one day when Mary noticed the little bump. It was a bluish mound under Sarah's skin, like a lump on a blueberry muffin. Then she noticed several other spots, all the same. They just weren't there a day before.

"Hon, would you come and look at this?" she called. Pete came into the baby's room and looked where Mary pointed. He didn't know what to think.

"Why don't you call Dr. Friedman? She'll know if it's anything important." So Mary called, and her pediatrician suggested an early appointment for the next morning. *Better to check it out,* the doctor said. *Hard to say over the phone.* But the baby was happy and fed well, so Mary was not particularly worried.

"Do you want me to take the day off and go with you?" Pete offered. She thought it sweet of him, but Mary declined. He had already missed so much work when the baby was born.

She went to the pediatrician's office by herself that day. As soon as Naomi Friedman saw the blue lumps under the skin, she frowned and started to probe around the rest of Sarah. She examined her for a long time, feeling deep in her abdomen.

"Mary, it's good that you noticed these so fast. That's always good. But that's not all that there is. There's a mass deep in her belly, near her kidney that I can feel."

"Mass? Are you talking about cancer?"

"Possibly. First I want to do a few tests in our lab. But then I'll be sending you over to the university hospital. Would you like me to call Pete? Do you want him to be there when we talk?"

221

"Yes, thank you." She held Sarah and nursed her while waiting for Pete. The baby nipped at Mary's breast playfully, not seeming to know there was anything wrong as her mother began to pray.

When Pete arrived, they drove together to the hospital. It was in the elevator to the children's floor that Mary first met Martha. On the same day that Teddy started his treatment on the school-age ward, baby Sarah began the fight for her life.

The six months of treatment began. One of the nurses came into the conference room to talk to me. "You need to talk to Mary. All the other mothers have learned to do the catheter care, but she seems to be on another planet. I don't think she is ever going to get it."

We had progressed so much in the treatment of these children that we had passed on much of the daily care to the mothers. Most of them, like Martha, seemed to like the responsibility. I went (as ordered) but heard another voice inside the room. I waited in the hall.

"I don't know why they expect that every mother will be Dr. Mom overnight," Mary's voice could be heard through the open door. "I'm just plain mom and never pretended to be anything else." She was talking to Martha.

"Here, let me show you how I do it," Martha offered. She set up the dressing kit very professionally and then showed Mary her personal little tricks.

"Well, maybe I can." Mary was encouraged.

"You've got it! See, I told you that you could do it," Martha triumphed.

When I heard her voice in the room, I knew that I did not need to talk to Mary. Martha was our parent pro. Mary would get it now. Twice Martha visited her at home, and they changed the dressing together. Martha seemed to be a natural when it came to working things out.

❦

Six months later, Teddy and Sarah were in the chemo room at the same time. "I don't know what the holdup is," Martha worried to the nurse. "His counts were ready long ago. Why isn't the chemo here yet?"

"That's okay, Mom," interjected Teddy, mesmerized by a Ninja Turtle video he was watching. "I'm in no hurry."

"I wish you wouldn't watch that trash," Martha complained to her son. "I brought tapes for you to listen to on your Walkman. Try to visualize your white cells fighting your tumor. Think positive thoughts."

"Sometimes it's not very positive having cancer, Mom. In fact, it stinks!" He still looked like an ordinary little boy, but in six months, Teddy seemed to have aged sixty years.

"Now if you could just channel all that anger against your tumor, you just might beat it," Martha scolded him.

"The only channel I'm interested in today is the Disney Channel. Let's not get too serious about all this business, Mom. You're not the one getting the chemo. This chemo is the best that anyone has. If it doesn't work, it's nobody's fault. It's not your fault or mine."

That was the point at which I had walked into the room. It was Teddy's last few words that caught my attention. *Nobody's fault*. I was worried about Martha. She held herself responsible for the lives and living of all she loved.

If the tumor came back, would she see it as her fault for not having researched enough? Or Teddy's fault because he preferred Ninja dudes to guided imagery? Or my fault because everyone likes to blame doctors today? Most likely, she would blame herself.

The problem was that the tumor *was* back. The reason for the delay in his chemo was a call I placed to the clinic from the Radiology Department. I told the nurse to hold the drugs. Despite everything we had offered Teddy, despite everything Martha had done, the neuroblastoma was back.

In bed that night, Pete sensed Mary's preoccupation. "Is something the matter, Hon? You seem to be in another world. Did something happen with Sarah today at the hospital?"

"It isn't Sarah. It's Teddy." She put down her prayer journal on the bedside table. For six months, every night, she had prayed over every family she met in our clinic. Each family had its own page. She was not the type to make a big issue of her beliefs publicly, but she was faithful in her private commitment to everyone she met.

"His tumor is back," Mary continued. "His mom took the news very hard. Teddy had to reassure Martha, promise her that he would fight it. I heard him talking to Dr. Komp afterward. He already knew before the X-ray was taken. All week he's been having pain in his arm. He knew what it meant, but he didn't say anything."

"There's nothing you can do for Martha," Pete interjected.

"She's talking about taking Teddy to another cancer center for an experimental treatment she heard about from another mother. She didn't even tell the doctors that. I heard her telling Teddy. The poor kid said, 'But Mom, I like it here. These people are my friends.' She blew up at him, 'This is your life we're talking about!' It wasn't a very pleasant scene."

"It's the strangest thing." Mary nestled to her husband, comforted by the familiar. "I had the feeling that she was angry with me, as if it were my fault. She asked me how Sarah is doing, and I was afraid to tell her that we had a good report.

"They started the same time, Sarah and Teddy. Martha has learned everything possible about neuroblastoma, followed his blood counts so carefully. And I never did any of that and Sarah is okay."

"Seems to me," said Pete, pulling her closer to him, "that there was a time that you accepted the responsibility for everything and everybody. When we first met, the entire Holocaust was your fault because your Uncle Hugo served in the *Luftwaffe*. Then it was the American Indians. They buried your heart at Wounded Knee."

Mary poked him in the ribs, "Come on! I don't even take the responsibility for your dirty socks anymore. I just leave them where you throw them until you trip over them or can't find any more to wear.

"But it's hard for someone like Martha," Mary continued. "She's always been so efficient and competent. Her house was always immaculate. Since Teddy's been sick, she realizes that she can't take care of the whole world alone, not even the people close to her."

"What's happening with her and Roger?" Pete asked. "I met him once at Candlelighters, and we just didn't connect. I was able to find something in common with all the other men, but Rog and I didn't seem to have mutual interests. He seemed to hide himself in his work when Teddy got sick. He just wanted to talk about insurance claims."

Pete's comment reminded Mary of a new concern. "Today when Dr. Komp told her the news, I asked Martha if she wanted to call Roger. I offered to stay with Teddy while she called. She just shook her head and got teary-eyed. She and Teddy looked at each other funny."

The first week after his relapse, Teddy got by with simple Tylenol, but then the pain accelerated and he reached the point he was at when the tumor was first found. Martha heard him crying in the night, awakening from her sleep. She turned toward Roger, forgetting that he was gone. It had been two months since he lived at home with them.

What hurt most was learning that Roger was already involved with another woman before Teddy became sick. As long as he had his perfect home and orderly life, he could tolerate his marriage. But cancer had changed all that, and he did not like the change. He blamed it all on Martha. This other relationship was undemanding, far simpler.

Martha went to Teddy's room and measured out the morphine to give him. She rocked him as it started to work its effect. She fell asleep with her child in her arms.

There was a knock at the door, late that night. The dream was so real that Martha told herself in her dream that this was no dream. She got up—in her dream—and went down to answer the door. At her front door was a carpenter, dressed in bib overalls with tools hanging from his waist. He held a lantern that was so bright that he seemed surrounded by light. But the light did not blind Martha nor hurt her eyes.

The carpenter told Martha that her house needed fixing and that he had come to repair it. She need not fear, for he would put her house in order. She should simply rest. In this dream that seemed no dream, Martha surrendered herself to the deep, peaceful gift of sleep. In the morning, she woke with Teddy in her arms.

The child whimpered slightly when she touched him. She reached for another dose of morphine as she kissed him on the forehead. "It's okay, Teddy," she murmured. "We're going to the hospital. Like you said, they're your friends there. They'll take care of the pain."

The next few days were crisis days for Teddy. Despite the morphine and chemotherapy, the tumor seemed to be progressing. He started bleeding from his stomach, and we couldn't seem to stop it. We transferred him to Intensive Care. The clinic nurses came to visit him there. He and Martha were among their favorites.

All the other mothers knew about Teddy. There is always a slight sense of guilt when your own child is doing well and another woman's son is dying, but everyone understood the common pain of belonging to the same family.

But there was another overwhelming pain that Martha must face in her unextended family. Teddy's hospitalization brought her and Roger back into daily contact. Because of the child that they both loved, they could not avoid facing each other across Teddy's bed. Together, they began to face that other pain.

Mary was there with Sarah as well the day that Teddy went to the ICU. Sarah was to be admitted for her last course of chemotherapy. A "coming off" party had been planned for the final day, a rite of passage.

When Sarah was settled in, Mary went to the Hunan Wok and brought food back to the ICU. Mary and Martha sat there eating silently, not even tasting the spicy meat. It was Martha who broke the silence in an uneven staccato.

"Do you know how much I resented you all these months? I'm ashamed to admit it. I even thought I hated you."

"Hush," said Mary, taking Martha into her arms. "You didn't really mean it. I know that." The tears were overflowing, and Martha let them wash out her pain.

"The worst day of all was the day that Teddy relapsed. I hated you that you never seemed to work at being the mother of a child with cancer and yet Sarah was doing well. She was even going to finish up her chemotherapy. How I hated you!"

Mary held Martha in her arms and rocked with her. I found them there together an hour later. There was unity and symmetry all at once in the pose, for were they not each a part of the other, a member of every mother? And both a part of me.

Late that night I returned to see a new patient in the Emergency Room. This child and her family were now settled in on the school-age floor. Tomorrow would be a big day for them and me. Before leaving for home, I stopped by to check on the rest of my brood.

Sarah slept quietly in her crib, Mary bedded down beside her. She was four days away from completing her treatment. Teddy also slept peacefully in the ICU, a grinning Garfield enfolded in his arms. In the side room where parents hold vigil, I found Martha and Roger, woven together, sleeping on a single cot.

I closed the door quietly to head home. Mary's daughter was on the homestretch. Martha's son was stable. And there were only a few hours left for me to sleep before the new day would begin.

3

Tamar's Touch

Tamar put ashes on her head, and tore the long robe that she was wearing; she put her hand on her head, and went away crying aloud as she went. Tamar remained, a desolate woman, in her brother Absalom's house.

2 SAMUEL 13:19,20 (NRSV)

Today some might call Carter Lowell a nerd. A longish mane spilled over his horn-rimmed glasses when he concentrated, forming a blond blind. Significant passages of his textbooks were punctuated by a sideways whiplash, a toss of head and neck to clear his vision. Book-bent was the common posture of this passionate scholar I knew years ago.

Although his school did not encourage accelerated progression, Carter had already skipped two grades by the time he reached the seventh. He was intrigued by the physical sciences. There was a lab in the corner of his bedroom, filled with beakers and Bunsen burners, flasks and flames. He continued to experiment long past school hours. *Excellent!* That was one of Carter's favorite phrases.

The boy was not one of those family surprises, more brilliant than his forebears. Both his parents had earned advanced degrees from prestigious institutions. He was clearly their child.

Carter was conceived when his mother was in graduate school. The boy's father was a post-doc who was one of her laboratory teaching assistants. Married to another woman, he returned to England with his wife when the boy was born.

When the nurse first handed the newborn baby to her, Tamara was afraid to touch him for fear that he would break. He was so tiny! She was so inexperienced. Tamara dropped out of grad school to move back with her parents and care for the child. Carter never knew his father.

Eventually she went back to complete her degree, and by the time I met her, Tamara Lowell was a well-established research scientist. The boy grew up mostly in the care of his grandparents.

There was a spirit in the lad that seemed alien in that particular family. He often felt as if he was a disappointment to them, especially to his mother. He didn't know how to please her. There was a warmth in Carter that was missing in his mother, an anticipation that something exciting might happen when you meet ordinary people.

Carter Lowell followed a solitary path. He walked alone to school each day. He ate alone in the lunchroom; he joined the math team rather than take up a sport. He didn't have a girlfriend, nor had he ever attended a school dance. Carter excelled in academics but lived on the fringes of teenage society. Younger than his classmates by two years, he had no real chums at school. To them, Carter seemed somewhat pompous. The poor kid was simply so enthusiastic about learning that he had no discern-

ment of when to remain silent in the presence of dolts. At sixteen, his passion was for Bach, not rock.

It was a distracting pain in his shoulder that brought
Carter to my office. The X-rays confirmed his family doctor's
suspicion of a bone tumor. In all my years of practice, I've
never had a conversation with a mother like that first session
when I told Dr. Lowell that Carter had cancer.

With anger flashing in her eyes, Tamara raged, "We
don't believe in God!" At that point in my life, neither did I,
but there was such a hatred in her voice that I took sharp
notice. I disbelieved quietly. There was a chilling intonation
to Tamara's denunciation. This was her first thought when I
told her that her son had cancer.

In those days, few teenagers with Ewing's sarcoma survived. Yet there were patients outliving our gloom-and-doom
talk every day. I wanted to talk about treatment. Tamara wanted
to talk about her son's death, there in that first meeting.

"How do patients with this tumor usually die?" she
asked as her son listened, tears running down his face. I could
not believe what I was hearing.

"It's possible that Carter may not die from this at all,"
I said. "We have treatment to offer. He may kick it rather than
succumb to it."

"There won't be a service," his mother continued.
"Not even an obituary in the papers. There is no life after
death." It was at that point that I realized that I had never
before met a parent of a child with cancer who actually
claimed to be an atheist.

I asked about the boy's father, if he would be coming
to see his son. The father, she said, was not a factor in his life
and would hardly be a help in his death.

Months into his treatment, Carter's English teacher noticed a constant sadness and asked if he would like to talk to a counselor. In a brief conversation, the school psychologist learned enough to alarm him. He called Tamara to suggest formal therapy. The notion was hostilely rejected. The boy simply lacked discipline, she said. His grandfather would speak to him.

His grandfather did talk to him once, during early puberty when Carter began to masturbate compulsively. He threatened to cut off both of the boy's hands if he ever did it again.

Eventually, Carter's sadness worked its way to the surface. He stole a car and crashed it into a telephone pole, nearly killing himself in the process. The juvenile court set psychotherapy as a condition for probation. Tamara had no other choice.

I liked Carter very much. He was quite pleasant, downright fun. He was intrigued by everything to do with his treatment. As a future scientist, he had to know all the technical points. He made me draw a schema of all the metabolic pathways, showing him the mechanism of action of every drug he would receive. He would study my charts for hours and then propose a new type of chemotherapy that might work better.

As independent as teenagers are, they treasure the comfort of a mother's hand or hug. They are rarely too proud in such circumstances to relinquish their hard-won control. Carter would have done the same. His mother rarely came into the treatment room while he was having a painful test or treatment. Tamara would not touch him.

Once he cried for her, and she fled the room. I held him in my arms as he wept silently for half an hour. When his tears were spent, he thanked me and left with Tamara. They walked down the hallway together without a word.

I must admit that I did not spend as much time with Carter as with my other patients. I struggled to treat this family in a nonjudgmental fashion but found it at times overwhelmingly difficult. I could not steel myself to spend any more time with them than was absolutely necessary. Carter sensed that, I think, and for that I've always had regret.

There was something in his mother's attitude that I could not understand. She seemed unable to affirm him as other mothers cherish their cancer-afflicted children. I wanted Carter to cry out, *Deliver me from this woman!* But of course, he didn't. He was her son, and he loved her dearly.

One day a minor surgical procedure caused him a great deal of pain. Carter cried for his mother. She raged at him and told him to act like a man. But she called him "Robbie," then left the room. I asked Carter, "Is 'Robbie' your middle name?"

"No. Robbie was my uncle. I never met him. He died before I was born."

The foreboding I had about this family would not go away. It was not for many years, long after Carter died, that I learned Tamara's story.

Tammy was a beautiful child, sired by a distant father. She was the only girl in the family, the youngest child. As a three-year-old, she passed long hours standing before her mirrored closet, choosing her dress for the day. She longed for her father to notice her.

It was her oldest brother who paid her the most attention. He became her hero, played with her when the others told the little kid to take off. He liked war games, tommy guns, and such. On his wall was a poster of Attila the Hun. When

Tammy got into fights, it was Robbie who fought her battles. She loved to come to his room to play.

She was six and he was fourteen when it started, one of those times she came to his room. No one else was home. She was pleased when he drew her close and set her on his lap. He rocked her and closed his eyes, rubbing her against him.

The first time he took her hand and asked her to touch him, she drew away. That's where boys were different from girls, what Mommy called their private parts. "It's okay, Tammy," he said, taking her hand again. "Don't I take care of you? I wouldn't do anything to hurt you. It will just be our secret. If you want to come to my room and play, then we will have our little secret."

The child loved her brother more than anyone in the world. The thought that he might not play with her was more than she could bear. And so she touched him where he asked. He held her hand, showed her how to please him. She was frightened when he groaned and seemed to be in another world. She tried to let go, but he held her hand tightly and kissed her.

That first night she had a nightmare and cried out in her sleep. As her mother came to comfort her, she found Robbie already in the hallway. "That's okay, Mom. I'll take care of her. I'll stay with her until she falls back asleep." And so, he held her and rocked her, and she was glad that he was there.

These trysts continued for three years. It was their secret, and he never hurt her, just showed her how to make him happy. And yet, the child had a sense of guilt and abandonment. Sometimes she wished that her parents would find out so that it would end. She felt dirty, yet she loved Robbie so much that she could not say no when he asked her to touch him in that special way.

It ended one night when Robbie came to her room. Their mother heard noise and went to check on Tammy. She screamed out and was quickly joined by her husband who throttled the boy, then slapped him hard in the face. Tammy pleaded for them not to hurt him, that it was her fault, not his. Robbie ran out of the house, grabbing the car keys on the way. His father screamed after him, "You're not my son. I disown you, you little piece of filth!"

The police did not identify Robbie until the next morning. Two patrol cars pursued him in a high-speed chase after they saw him driving 120 miles an hour down the highway.

The car caught fire as soon as it hit the telephone pole. They had to wait for the wreckage to cool before they could check the motor number against vehicle records. No identification was found on the body or in the car. The police considered it fortunate that it was a single-car accident, that no one but the driver was killed.

There was no service for Robbie, no obituary in the newspaper. The small-town headlines had already said more than enough. The parents explained to friends that the body was burned beyond recognition. It was simpler to have a private graveside service. They just set him in the ground without a marker.

Tammy was not there to see her brother committed to the earth. She was sobbing in her room, blaming herself for her brother's death. If she had not touched him, Robbie would never have died.

When her son was three years old, Tamara first noticed that Carter looked like her brother. By the time he was six years old, she found the likeness intolerable. From that time on, she never touched her son. That is, until the week of his death.

I suppose it was inevitable that Carter never did well. He faced death less than a year after his tumor was first discovered. To help with his pain, to try for another remission, we gave Carter more powerful chemotherapy. His pain was controlled, but an infection developed that caused his fever to climb.

Two teary-eyed nurses tried to restrain the boy onto a cooling blanket as his temperature and his body soared. They held his outstretched arms as I heard him cry out, "Oh God, tell me if you exist." Seven lasting words.

Can a woman forget her nursing child, or show no compassion for the child of her womb? Somehow, there had to be an answer for this almost motherless child's needs. If there was a God, surely he would reach out in mercy to this young man.

I never knew what brought the change in Tamara and most likely never will. It was simply that all of a sudden she seemed to be freed to meet her son's needs. She took Carter home.

I visited them as often as possible. Although his body was deteriorating, the boy was at peace. I sat on his bed one day, still holding his hand after I finished checking his pulse, extending a medical touch into a more human one.

From his bed we could see some ducks climbing out of a pond and padding up onto a tennis court. Two neighbor boys were volleying with more vigor than skill that day. There was longing in Carter's eyes, a tiny benign spark of envy. But then he closed his eyes as if to blink them away and himself back to this room.

Carter thought that his temperature was going up again, and he was right. Tamara came quietly into the room,

236

laid her hand on his forehead, confirmed his suspicion. Then she took a cool cloth and wiped her son's face. I moved away from the bed to see what would happen next.

She took a basin of water and a cloth, began to wash his body, then spread baby oil on his shoulders. The muscles relaxed, the body did not arch. Carter fell asleep, gently holding his mother's hand to his lips. Her own lips met her son's hand gently before releasing it.

Tamara walked with me to my car. I could think of nothing to say. There was not much to discuss, medically speaking. All my unanswered questions were far too personal to pursue. I took my questions home with me, leaving Carter in his own bed, with his own family.

On the way back to the hospital, I remembered Carter's prayer to the God in whom his mother did not believe and an ancient promise as well: *Even if a mother were to forget, yet I will not forget you. Perhaps,* I thought, *there is a God who hears the prayers of the poor and afflicted. If there is a Creator of this universe, surely he must be generous enough to tell one dying boy, "Yes, I exist. And I love you."*

After Carter's death, at home, there was a notice in the local newspaper. A memorial service would take place by the duck pond he could see from his window. Carter deserved to be honored and remembered, it said. He was Tamara Lowell's beloved son.

4

Hannah's Exultation

They brought the child to Eli. And [Hannah] said, "Oh, my lord!... I am the woman who was standing here in your presence, praying to the LORD. For this child I prayed; and the LORD has granted me the petition that I made to him. Therefore I have lent him to the LORD; as long as he lives, he is given to the LORD."

1 SAMUEL 1:25–28 (NRSV)

She sat quietly in the waiting room reading *Family Circle*. Farm fresh, Hannah wore no makeup. Her sun-streaked hair was plaited into a single French braid. Until she looked up, there was nothing remarkable to note. But she did look up, filling the room with light as you beheld her eyes—striking green. Hannah looked back down at her magazine and blended back into the shadows.

She sat in the waiting area, dressed in blouse and jeans, no different from other mothers in the room. Yet I realized that that was exactly what distinguished her the most. Where was the freshly pressed dress or tasteful suit? Blue jeans are for later, battle fatigues for vets. Sammy was a new patient, but his mother dressed like an old-timer.

This was my image of Hannah when we first met and every time thereafter. If she was anxious about our first visit, I couldn't tell it from her face or clothes. As circumstances changed, Hannah integrated without compromising, accommodated without conceding. When I walked into the waiting area to call them, Sammy was playing on the floor beside her. She allowed her five-year-old son to play, undisturbed. She neither hovered over him nor gathered him to her arms.

Like his mother, the child seemed at peace. And yet, I knew that their pediatrician had told Hannah his worst fears. There was a lump the size of a golf ball growing rapidly in Sammy's neck. He had been hospitalized nearer to home for many weeks, treated with antibiotics. Now it was time for him to see a cancer specialist for children. Hannah knew why she was there. And so did Sammy.

I've seen her face and his in my imagination so often that time does not seem to diminish the clarity of the picture. There was something about the triad we formed—Hannah, Sammy, and I—that drew us together those many years ago. It is not an easy thing to define.

Long ago, we put aside a distance that was never meant to be. Hannah and I were closer than sisters. We were like mother and mother to the same child. It was a mark of her deep trust that she was willing to share her son with me. Sammy helped close the distance the first day.

When I walked with them to an examining room, he looked up at me shyly. Sammy ran his hand through his freshly punked hair and sighed, and with the sigh, sucked in on his cheeks, deepening his dimples. There were flecks of gold in the green that sparkled when the light hit his irises, flickered from his eyes to mine and back to the diamond earring in his left earlobe. Finally, he tittered a little boy's titter, and Hannah prodded him. "Well, aren't you gonna ask her?"

"Ask me what?" I was intrigued by the family secret, the covert glance that leaped and rebounded from boy to mom to boy. *Whatever it was must be worth knowing*, I thought.

Sammy cupped his mouth to my ear, whispered moistly into it, "Can I have your autograph?" I stood bolt upright, startled by his question.

"My autograph? Nobody's ever asked me for my autograph before! I am so honored."

"Patty said you're real famous."

Hannah quickly explained that Patty was his favorite nurse. She was the one who stayed with him in the Intensive Care Unit when he was most frightened. Just one week earlier, Sammy was discharged from that hospital and now was coming to another. He was afraid to come to a big hospital, and his nurse had calmed his fears in the best way she could imagine.

"You're going to see *Dr. Komp?*" she asked him. "Why, she's so famous!" Sammy was impressed. Next to his mother, Patty was the most important woman in the world. And now, I seemed fortunate enough to be joining that short list of feminine luminaries.

I fetched a reprint of an article I had published and signed it for Patty. Then I gave Sammy a publicity photograph that I found in my desk, and I autographed it regally. He was smitten.

The child went to the lab for his blood work with the photo pressed to his chest. He showed it to each technician he could find. They all told him that I had never given any of them an autographed photo. He blushed with pleasure. I was blushing, too. The blood-flush in our cheeks, Sammy's and mine, sealed our kinship.

Sammy never really responded well to treatment. Nothing we could offer would eradicate the errant clone of cancer that defied the best we had. After our first meeting, there were few days that he was in his own home. We tried to send him out on pass a few times so that he could visit his puppy and sleep in his own bed.

Each day, Hannah saw me walk softly into another child's room, suspecting the reason for my uncharacteristic solemnity. Every week, she read other mothers' tears, sensed the parting of their sons and daughters. There were no secrets on a children's ward. Wordlessly, mysteries were shared.

She played music for Sammy, there in the hospital. One day he heard these words: *Our God is an awesome God. He reigns from heaven above with wisdom, power and love.* The words enkindled his imagination.

"You're kidding, Mom!" he said. "God is awesome?"

Hannah thought about it, then answered with great confidence, "Sure!"

"God is *awesome?*" he repeated. "Does God wear an earring?"

"Well," thought Hannah, "he would if he wanted to!"

"Awesome!" was her little one's response.

I watched Hannah watch us. Many a time when we made rounds, she stood close, listening carefully to our medical chatter. She appeared more a part of our team than an outsider to the medical mystery. This was her son, after all. Hannah was not to be shut out.

During his illness, the disease filled Sammy's brain. First it robbed him of his speech, next of his vision, finally of his ability to walk. Never have I felt as frustrated as when that tumor progressed, robbing Sammy of everything that we prize about being human. And yet, Sammy maintained a serenity that was beyond explanation. He could barely move but did what he could without complaint. He could finger his little yellow tape recorder and play his awesome tape.

He was in a room with three other brain-damaged boys, worse off than he, if such was possible. One child had fallen out of a fourth-story window. Another had been beaten. The third was the hapless victim of a hit-and-run driver. The room was a vegetable garden, filled with wilting young life. Mothers sat patiently at their sides, encouraging their sons with their therapy, hoping and praying for a miracle.

The dimples in his steroid-plumped cheeks were flattened out, altering his smile. Sammy used the little strength he had in his right hand to operate his tape recorder. Hannah and I chatted on, discussing his latest test results. From time to time, we would look over to Sammy. He had lain back and listened to his music with the volume turned down so as not to disturb others in the room.

As we spoke, we heard a blast of song: *We declare that the kingdom of God is here! The blind see, the deaf hear, the lame man is walking. Sicknesses flee at his voice. The dead live again and the poor hear the good news. Jesus is King, so rejoice!* We were startled, as were the others in the room but we all heard the words.

Without being asked, Sammy turned down the volume when that song was finished. He continued to listen quietly to the other songs. Then, with the little strength that he had in the tips of his fingers, he rewound the tape. He played it quietly until he reached the same song.

We declare that the kingdom of God is here . . . Again, the blind, the deaf, and the lame in that room were startled to attention. It was obvious that Sammy knew what he was doing. I went to the side of his bed and took his hand. He smiled his sunny smile.

"You really believe that, don't you, kiddo?" I asked. And he nodded vigorously. Sammy believed. But did I? In his childlike faith, this six-year-old found comfort in these words. No, *more than comfort*. He seemed to find peace and meaning for his life. But his apparent peace brought anxious thoughts into my own mind.

What would Sammy think of his awesome God if he was not healed? Surely the prophet meant spiritual blindness, not physical. Then I realized that the fears were mine and mine alone. *Truly I tell you, unless you change and become like children, you will never enter the kingdom of heaven.* It was my God who was too small. Sammy and his awesome God shared the secret of his peaceable kingdom.

The child was transferred to the Intensive Care Unit and kept my beeper ringing busily when I was at home. While he was in the hospital, there were very few quiet evenings.

It was such a day one Sunday when I took out a few hours to teach my junior-high-school Sunday school class. Thirty-two rascals kept my focus on life, and I used my guitar like a mighty weapon. As long as I could keep them singing, I was in control and we were all happy. Then my beeper went off. I left the class for a few minutes to use the phone in the pastor's study. When I returned, they sat there silently, waiting for me to say something.

What could I say? What could they or should they understand about a child younger than they, clinging to life on a respirator? I felt their eyes on me as I sat down. The children anticipated that I might need prodding, so they had elected a representative, a doctor's daughter. "Did somebody die?" she asked.

Fool that I was, I did not even realize that the children knew what type of doctor I was. Did healthy pubescents even know what it meant to be a "pediatric oncologist"? My innocence and theirs were lost that day together. As carefully as I could, I told them about Sammy. They continued to stare and wait. It was clear that they were looking for more than a story. So I suggested that we pray for Sammy, together.

After church, I went to the hospital and spoke with Hannah. I told her about the children, how they had challenged me, how we had prayed together, how I had again learned to never, never again underestimate a child.

Several days later, Sammy died. I stood at his bedside, silent and saddened. Hannah handed me a letter. It was for my Sunday school class. In it, she thanked the children for their prayers and told them that God had indeed answered their prayers. *The dead live again. Jesus is King, so rejoice!* Sammy was with his awesome God.

❧

I've thought about our first meeting often. Long after I knew Hannah well, I kept replaying that waiting room scene, imagining what she was thinking as she waited for me to call out Sammy's name.

I recalled her face at Sammy's bedside in the ICU as I primed myself to deliver the latest grim news. But she was at peace. Each visit, she smiled at me gently and inquired, "How are you this morning?" This woman was a gift.

She looked just the same that day at his funeral, except for the dark dress and the tears that filled her eyes when she saw me. I walked to the chapel, weeping myself. And yet, as we embraced, it was not for herself alone that she wept. She wept for me as well.

"Oh, Diane, I'm so sorry. You lose so many children. I wanted to give you one child who would live. I wanted Sammy's life to be a gift to you."

As long as I had known her, I still was stupefied. What type of woman was this who could lose her son and grieve for the loss that another woman might feel for the same child?

In some sense, Sammy was never fully Hannah's, simply hers on loan. How could this young mother fathom what it was like for me, a middle-aged childless woman, to "mother" other women's children and lose so many? I hardly knew, myself, and yet she seemed to know.

Hannah visited the hospital often after Sammy's death. The bonds that tied us were too strong for death to sever. Often, one or more of her younger children came along. Hannah never shut them out of this part of her life while Sammy lived, and she would not exclude them now.

Little Amy seemed particularly pleased to come back each time, as if she were in a place where Sammy still lived. As young as she was, she thought of us as people who loved and cared for her brother. Our "home" was a safe place where she could freely speak of Sammy.

These visits always pleased me, bringing a welcome break to a day's drudgery. Although her son was gone, our journey together was not yet complete. After seeing Hannah, it was easier for me to face a newer mother. It was on one of these occasions, with Amy at her side, that she sought to speak to me privately.

"I've never told you this before. The day that Sammy died, he said something that told me that he knew that the end had come. He said, 'I want to go home.' The nurses thought he meant home to Lovingston, but I knew what he really meant. I knew that he knew that this earth was never his real home."

Years had passed since Sammy's death. You could no longer speculate that she was operating on the emotional high that often surges after a loss. She was so calm, so radiant. I had the sense of being on holy ground, speaking to someone who knew what it means to love her child with her whole heart but to love God more.

Hannah wasn't looking at me as she was speaking. Her gaze was on another time and place as she exulted, "I was there when he was born. I was there when he went home. It was such a privilege to be his mother. I am so blessed." And so was I.

5

Elena's Prayer

The daughter of Pharaoh came down to bathe at the river.... She saw the basket among the reeds.... When she opened it, she saw the child. He was crying, and she took pity on him.

EXODUS 2:5–6 (NRSV)

She sat in a cornfield, transfixed by the blue morning mist that enfolded the distant volcano. There were rumors that the *judiciales* had come, searching for guerrillas in the highlands of Guatemala. It was hard to believe that such a beautiful land could be so violent. Elena sighed and replaced her flat basket on her head before she headed home to the shack.

They caught her as soon as she entered the room. Her youngest sister was cowering in a corner, sobbing. Her eyes followed the child's animal-wild gaze. Their mother lay motionless on the floor, bloodied, naked, disemboweled. Elena spun around to see one of the *militares* drag her brother into the room. His eyes were swollen shut, his mouth filled with blood. There was a gun to his head, and he was sobbing.

The soldiers had raped their mother before they murdered her. Now it was Elena's turn. One of the *militares*, big-bellied, with rotten teeth and pig-sweating face, reached down to undo his trousers. In less than a bloody minute, he rolled off her, leaving her dress stained, reeking of his brief presence.

Elena lay there unmoving, afraid that he might start all over again. Instead, his *companeros* took his place, one after the other, all night. She tried to imagine herself far away from this pathetic village with its tin-roofed shanties, away from a land bent on annihilating its entire Indian population. A soldier slapped her so hard that her body went crashing into the *bajareque* wall and she lost consciousness. Her eyes stared up, vacantly; blood poured from her mouth. Despite their intentions, she survived. The next day she awoke to find her mother, father, three sisters, and two brothers dead and mutilated. All because her father was an *indio*.

Fearing that the soldiers would return, Elena fled with the little food she could find. They had stolen their few miserable chickens. She wrapped her provisions in her basket and herself with a shawl for protection from the night air as she crept deep into the highlands.

When her food ran out, she stole at night from village to village. It was a mark of the poverty in that region that there was so little garbage to be found. Very rarely, there was a slow-moving scrawny chicken to snatch. It was frightening at night, alone in the mountains, but she feared the animals less than the human predators who might find her hiding place. She kept on the move in the highlands to avoid being spotted by either the guerrillas or the federal troops.

At first she didn't know what was happening to her body, why her breasts were budding out, her belly swelling. But then she knew.

Her first reaction was to be ashamed, to hate what was in her that the soldiers had left behind. And yet, the child was also hers, part Indian. She would not let them wipe her people off the face of the earth. Elena might perish, but she swore that her baby would survive. And once it was born, she would find a way for the child to have a better life.

She thought of the few prayers she had heard the rare times that a priest came as far as their little village. Elena tried to remember what the angel said to Maria when she, young, yet unmarried, found herself pregnant. *The Lord is with you. Don't be afraid*. She struggled to recall Maria's response. *My soul magnifies the Lord, and my spirit rejoices in God my Savior*.

Every night, she fell asleep with those words on her lips and her tzute wrapped around her. She prayed that God would guard the baby that she carried. She wept for her murdered mother, mourned her loss. There was no one to explain to a young girl that which was happening to her body.

But what of Maria? Did she tell her own mother at first? How could she convince a pious family that she was pregnant by God? Her cousin Elizabeth believed the angel story that Maria told and shared her outrageous joy. That was what Elena prayed for—the gift of outrageous joy, the ability to bless her baby for the gift of its companionship. *God has looked with favor on the lowliness of his servant*.

It was at dawn when the pains began. Elena rocked herself, hidden in another cornfield. She focused on the same distant volcano, allowing field and mist to midwife her. She dared not cry out lest she be found. As if to parrot her pangs, a bright orange glow erupted through the mist, crowning the volcano. With each pain, she remembered that other young woman who was far from home when her own time came. *The Lord is with me!* was Maria's exclamation. *Maria's Son, Jesus, stay with me!* Elena prayed as a molten river snaked its way down the volcano, and her little daughter burst into the world.

She named the baby *Gabriella* after Maria's angelic visitor. She held the infant to her hunger-flattened breast and was amazed at the strength with which the baby sucked. The mother was wasting away, but the baby was fat. Elena might not survive, but the infant was sturdy and fighting for life.

There was no moon or stars that night to guide her as she left the *altiplano* for the city far below. She heard the treacherous racing waters in the deep ravine below as she descended from the highlands and made her way to the city.

She left the baby in the basket on the steps of a church, snugly wrapped in her shawl. Certain that the nuns would find it quickly, she stole back to the highlands, unprotected from the night air. *Maria's Son, Jesus, stay with my Gabriella*, she prayed as she collapsed to the ground. She had finished the task that had kept her alive all those months. There was a smile of incomparable joy on her lips as she surrendered to the chilling darkness.

It was the crying that woke Father Carrera. He stumbled out of his house next to the church and found a bright Indian cloth in motion. There was no one in sight—there rarely was when these babies were left. These villagers never seem to change, he thought. And there is no priest who will stay there and teach them a better way.

The last missionary was killed by the military when he tried to organize the peasants. These young priests all seem to get radical when they work in the highlands. Better for a priest to stay here in the squalor of the city. Just last week two nuns were raped and murdered while the soldiers forced a young seminarian to look on. They left the young man for dead, but now he is safely on his way back to Iowa where corn can be grown in more peaceful circumstances.

The baby continued to cry, so he lifted the basket and headed for the convent. The sisters were dwindling in number, but they would care for this baby. They had contacts in El Norte who seemed to find families who wanted these babies. If not, there was always the orphanage, already teeming with the orphans of the *desaperecido*, the "disappeared." But this one was a squaller! She would wake the whole city before the first rooster had anything to say about today.

Thousands of miles from the Guatemalan highlands, another mother was in labor. Tanya's husband was at her side for the birth of her first child. Sean would be there again with each pregnancy, holding her hand. Over the years they would be three times together in such a room. Only the first time did they take a baby home.

Their first child was named Elizabeth, a sunny Gerber baby sporting a wisp of blonde hair. She slept through the night from the second night on, this dream child. Then a year later, Christopher was born. He was a handsome boy-child with thick, black hair. But his liver and spleen were swollen, making him look painfully pregnant.

That was when I met Tanya and Sean for the first time. Just before Christopher died, we found a rare blood incompatibility. We knew that this condition would get worse with each child. There was no vaccine against this like the one available for "Rh babies." The young couple was distraught. How could a baby die so quickly?

But they were young and healthy and they still had Lizzy. Six months later, Tanya was pregnant again. This time, they stayed close to home, avoiding crowds and sick people. Perhaps Tanya had caught some virus, they thought, and passed it on to the baby. Better to play it safe.

Christopher's death had forewarned us, and for the next pregnancy the perinatal team was on standby. Everything went smoothly until the seventh month. My telephone rang when Tanya arrived in the OB suite. We tried to give the baby a blood transfusion while she was still in Tanya's womb, but labor started, and the mother was transferred to the Labor Room.

A nurse looked worried. After she saw the monitor, she left the room to call Dr. Kelly. Sean saw the moving, white line on the monitor and the digits flashing out above. He had seen enough of these machines to worry himself. His brow furrowed when he saw the number displaying the fetal heart rate. A baby's heart rate shouldn't be that slow. Tanya had another strong labor pain and gripped his hand. The baby's heart rate dropped even lower.

Dr. Kelly was in her blue scrubs when she came in. She, too, frowned when she saw the monitor. "Tanya, I think the safest thing to do is a Caesarean. That baby wants to come out as soon as possible, and I think we should help her."

Tanya nodded, and the nurse wheeled her toward the operating room. Sean squeezed her hand so tightly that it turned white. "Please, dear God, not again! It can't be. Not this early!"

Amanda, their third child, was born dead. Tanya and Sean could not believe it had happened again and might happen to future babies. How could this be? They were both healthy. They both wanted a large family. Why was this happening to them?

After Tanya was asleep in her hospital room, Sean went to his mother's home and took six-year-old Lizzy in his arms. "No baby, Daddy?" she asked. He didn't know what to say to his daughter. Tears filled his eyes. "Don't cry, Daddy," the child tried to console him. "It's okay. God will give us a baby. You'll see, Daddy. God has already made a baby for us to take care of."

❧

Tanya and Sean tried for years to adopt a baby. Their problem was that they had a living child. They would not be high up on an agency list. They called me once to ask me if I had any ideas, but I didn't. It was a frustrating time. But when they were sad, Lizzy would come and hold them close. "Don't cry. God has already made a baby for us. You'll see."

It was a friend who told them about special children who needed adoption. And soon they were talking to an agency about an older child, a seven-year-old girl, Lizzy's own age.

They came home to tell Lizzy and show her a picture. The child was as dark as their daughter was fair. But when she saw the picture, Lizzy lit up. "That's our baby! That's my new sister that God had already made for us. She looks like an angel!"

❧

They met Gabriella at the airport. She was accompanied by a nun from the convent orphanage. Gaby clung to the little woman shyly, amazed by all the new sights and sounds around her. It was Lizzy who went over to her first and put her arms around her.

"You're my sister. God sent you to us. We're going to take care of you. Everything is going to be all right. You'll see." She took the child's hand and led her over to Tanya and Sean, who hardly knew what to do except follow Lizzy's lead. They stood there embracing the two girls, weeping. When they looked up, the nun was gone. All the child's possessions were in a small bag woven with an Indian design. They took her small hand and brought Gabriella home.

Lizzy insisted on sharing a room with her new sister so that she wouldn't be afraid in the dark. She showed her every corner of the house, not the least bit concerned that Gaby spoke no English. She picked out her favorite doll and gave it to her new sister, her first gift.

After dinner they found Gaby at the window, looking out and weeping. That night in bed, she sobbed. Lizzy crawled into bed with her and held her in her arms. "Don't cry, Gaby. We love you. God sent you to us. You'll see." Lizzy would rock the child until she fell asleep. In the morning, Tanya and Sean would find them in bed together, intertwined.

At times Lizzy could be overwhelming. She was determined to teach her new sister everything that she knew. And Lizzy was a very bright little girl. She took out the family photo album. "This is Grandma and Grandpa Rhodes. You'll meet them at Christmas. Did you ever meet your grandparents? Do you even know who your mother was?" The chatter was constant. Although Tanya didn't think that Gaby understood a word, she was reassured by Lizzy's confidence about their new life together.

Every night, after supper, they would find Gaby by the window with tears in her eyes. And every night she would cry in her bed until Lizzy came and stilled her fears. Tanya and Sean started to worry. Most of all, they worried that Lizzy was taking on too much responsibility for a seven-year-old child.

Tanya called to ask if I could check Gaby out for medical problems. There were none to be found. I suggested contacting the orphanage of the Little Sisters of Jesus, where she had grown up, to ask if there was anything that the sisters recognized. The Mother Superior told them about the circumstances of the child's arrival.

Gaby was found on their doorstep, crying, and cried almost constantly for the next three months until a new sister came to their order. The only way the infant would sleep was to be rocked by Sister Maria, the nun who accompanied her on the flight to the United States. She could pacify the infant when no one or nothing else could.

When she was older, the child would sneak to the sister's room whenever she had night terrors, and they would find them in bed together in the morning. And yet it was Sister Maria who insisted that they must find a real home for her, that she should not grow up in an orphanage.

At Christmastime, Lizzy insisted that they dress alike. Lizzy carefully placed the photo of them, smiling together, in the album next to the pictures of the babies who no longer were alive, next to her own pictures as an only child. "God did not mean for me to be an only child," she would explain to Gaby. "Mommy and Daddy have so much love that it just wouldn't be fair. So God brought you to us so that you could be in our family album and we could love you."

The two girls would walk to school hand in hand and sit next to each other in the classroom. With Lizzy for a tutor, Gaby's English was coming along rapidly. Tanya and Sean decided to try separate rooms for the girls but abandoned that plan after three sleepless, sobbing nights. They asked Lizzy to try to sleep in her own bed, to help Gaby get used to sleeping alone.

One day, while cleaning, Tanya took out Gaby's Indian sack that came with her from the orphanage. In it she found a dog-eared photo of the nun, Sister Maria. She bought a small silver frame for it in a shop that day and placed it on Gaby's bedside table. When the child saw it that evening, she tore it out of the frame and held it to her, rocking and weeping. It was then that Tanya decided what she needed to do. She called the convent.

"Mother Superior," she began, "I know that this is a very unusual request. But I know that you want what is best for Gaby. She's still having problems adapting, and I think it would be a tremendous help if Sister Maria could come here and live with us for a while. I don't know what that will mean for her vows, but if there's a way, we promise that we'll help her however possible."

"You're right, Señora Rhodes, that is a most unusual request. Sister Maria is a most devout member of our order. She prays for all the unwanted and orphaned children of these villages. She devotes herself to the memory of the Holy Innocents."

"What's her story?" Tanya asked. "Do you know anything about the woman?"

"She's never told us, my child, and we have never asked. You must understand the sadness of the poor people who come to us. Forgive me for my impatience. These are trying times. We are here to be her family now. You are asking for her to leave her family."

"I just know that it's important to Gaby. Somehow I know your Sister Maria can help this one child even more than her prayers help all the other children. Can you trust a mother's heart? Do you understand what I'm trying to say?"

"I can only promise to pray about it. And ask the other sisters. That is all I can promise," came the answer.

"We'll be praying, too," said Tanya. "Please tell Sister Maria that we pray for her every day."

"Please pray for all of us," she murmured. Tanya heard exhaustion in the woman's voice. "These are difficult times for the peasants here. And when we try to help them, we ourselves must be ready to suffer and die."

It was Lizzy who decided that they should decorate the whole house to welcome Sister Maria. She went with Tanya to pick out curtains and a bedspread for the room where she would sleep. Lizzy insisted that she feel at home with them. Then Lizzy took Gaby's hand and led her over to the party favors to buy special balloons. Tanya had never seen Gaby so excited.

Tanya was sure they had made the right decision. And for Mother Superior, it evolved as an answer to prayer. Two more lay catechists in the region had been murdered by the death squads. The *militares* announced that the sisters must vacate the convent. It would become a command post for the federal troops.

Sister Maria would be assigned to the Rhodes as Gaby's nanny. She would continue with her prayers while the child was in school. In her heart, Mother Superior wished that Gaby and Sister Maria weren't the only ones to find a compassionate solution. She would bring the nun with her when she returned, defeated, to her order's mother house in New England.

At home, the children insisted on decorating the room themselves. Lizzy and Gaby blew up all the balloons and hung festive banners. Tanya was glad they had something to keep them out of mischief while she planned the welcome dinner. In three hours, Sister Maria would be at the Bradley Airport. Lizzy and Gaby closed the door behind them when they finished the room, wanting it to be a surprise. Tanya smiled.

The scene at the airport was what Tanya and Sean expected. The child ran to the nun and wouldn't let go of her.

They kept hugging and weeping, happily reunited. Gaby chattered away, hardly letting Sister Maria get a word in. She introduced the nun to Lizzy. Those were the only words Tanya and Sean understood. *My sister, Lizzy.*

Sister Maria was overwhelmed by their house. Their modest raised ranch seemed like a luxury villa to her. From the nun's face, Tanya knew that this was the right decision. She hoped that her order would let Sister Maria stay for a very long time. The children took her by the hand to show her to her room.

With great fanfare, the girls opened the door. The room was filled with balloons. Festooned across the wall over the bed was a large banner: WELCOME HOME, NITA.

"Lizzy," Tanya said. "Her name is Maria, not Nita."

"No, Mommy," answered the child. "Sister Maria is her religious name. Her real name is Elena. Her family always called her Elenita, little Elena. Gaby calls her Nita . . ."

6

Hagar's Flight

～━━ﾐ━━～

And God heard the voice of [Ishmael]; and the angel of
God called to Hagar from heaven, and said to her,
"What troubles you, Hagar? Do not be afraid; for God
has heard the voice of the boy where he is. Come, lift
up the boy and hold him fast with your hand, for I will
make a great nation of him."

Genesis 21:17–18(NRSV)

It was in a little grocery store run by a man from her
uncle's village that Hagar first saw him. She was sent by her
mother to buy red lentils, goat cheese, and fresh, flat Turkish
bread. He came in the crowded little shop in the Kreuzberg
section of Berlin with another man. He was a "guest worker"
as they called them. Newly arrived in Germany, he intended
to make his fortune in this wealthy Western land.

He was taller than the other men Hagar knew, her
father's friends. His eyes were a brighter brown and very direct.
When he looked at her, she looked down modestly. Hagar
wouldn't want him to guess her thoughts. But then, she really did.

The next time she saw him, he was in a café drinking thick Turkish coffee with three other men. The men were smoking and laughing when she spotted him. She kept her eyes down but noted that he saw her pass. His glance followed her all the way home. Hagar smiled secretly.

That evening, while the others slept, Hagar lay awake thinking about her future. Life in Ankara had been difficult. There was no work for her father there. True, the outskirts of Ankara were better than the small village where her cousins lived. But to Hagar, Berlin was pure luxury. She had seen how the Germans lived. Her mother worked as a maid for such a family. They were very polite with their maid but somewhat distant, to Hagar's way of thinking. At least, they were honest and fair.

Hagar learned a little of their language—more than her mother—from the children of this house. She looked around her family's tiny room and then thought about the grand flat in which her mother's employers lived. It seemed that these Germans worked hard, and that was how these possessions came to them. If she could only find a man who was a hard worker, someday she might live in luxury as well.

His name was Ibrahim. She heard his friend address him as she walked behind them on the street one day. She kept a slight distance so that he would not know she was there with her little brother. She wanted to learn everything she could about him.

He spoke with his friend of a new opportunity and high wages. There was a contractor looking for men newly arrived from Turkey. They would be rich within a short time. As she came close to her apartment building, she motioned to little Mustafah to run ahead. Then she ran after her brother, passing the men, yelling at the child in rapid-fire Turkish. She saw Ibrahim turn and note her entering the building. As she closed the door, she looked directly at him, and he nodded his respect.

It was the same evening that he came to talk with her father. The two men went to the local café and the nuptial negotiations began.

Her mother's employer found a job for the new bride with another family. Hagar was proud that she could contribute to their meager income. Her husband took all their earnings to send home to his impoverished family. Still, she hoped that one day they, too, would have a fine apartment.

It was springtime when her clothes fit too tightly. Her mother laughed, "Pray that Allah will send you a son. Then all will go well with your husband." So she did.

Ismael came into the world with a lusty scream that satisfied the midwife. Hagar was happy that she had given her husband a healthy son. Ibrahim was pleased with his son and tender with him and Hagar. But he spoke of returning to Turkey, to that tiny village far from the city life of Ankara.

Hagar was stunned with the news. From the moment her family arrived in Germany, she had never thought to return to the poverty she had known in Turkey. She stood on the train platform, a study in brown and gray. A two-tone kerchief covered her hair. The buttons of her mud-brown sweater strained to protect her from the cold. She gathered a plain gray coat around her to shield her from the wind that blew across her pregnant body.

What did wealth mean in a tiny village where Islamic custom supplanted federal regulations in everyday life? In Germany she had far more freedom than she had ever known before. What could she look forward to there? Hopefully, her second child would also be a boy. The father laughed and played with his son as Hagar watched her life pass from west to east.

Life was very difficult for Hagar in this village. Ibrahim's relatives treated her like a foreigner and criticized her Western ways. She gave birth to their second child, a daughter. For the next few years, daughter followed daughter. As his father had before him, Ibrahim took a second wife. She bore him three sons in as many years.

Some ten years after their return, Ibrahim developed a cough that racked his body at night. Hagar begged him to see a German-trained doctor in Ankara and traveled with him on a crowded bus. It broke down en route to the city, and they huddled together during the night as the driver waited for dawn to start the repairs. When dawn came, Ibrahim was dead.

After his death, Ibrahim's mother treated her like a servant. Hagar longed for her own mother and the prospect of a future for her son. She thought of how the German family had treated her. And at least they had paid her money for her menial work. So she and her children started back on the road to Ankara and from there to Germany. From these two hostile worlds, Hagar chose the lesser of the two evils.

Ten years later, Hagar's mother still spoke little German. Hagar scolded her mother, warned her that her own life would be better if she looked out for herself better. But her mother lashed back. Her daughter was a foreigner to her own people. And with so many fancy ideas! Who was the daughter to advise the mother? Life was not meant to be exciting, Hagar. We are only meant to survive.

She worked hard now to learn more German. Hagar determined that through education her children would find their way out of a ghetto existence and take their place among doctors, lawyers, and other learned ones.

They were back in Berlin for only two weeks when Ismael took ill. She fought the sense of panic rising biliously from the pit of her stomach. This could not be happening to her twice! He was her son, her sun, her hope. She meant for Ismael to grow up, to become a doctor, to make his way between the two worlds. It could not be happening to him. It was through Ismael that she would be vindicated.

It was a week later that she found herself with him in a doctor's office at the medical school. There, she read eyebrows instead of reports. Words can evade, even lie. Even if only briefly, the eyes must tell the truth. The nurses were gentle with her and treated her with respect, but the doctors confused her with too many words. In her head and heart, a voice screamed obscenities that drowned them out.

I met Hagar the morning after Ismael was admitted to the hospital. I was on sabbatical that year, visiting a children's cancer ward and my German counterparts. There seemed to be many Turkish children in this most Western of European countries.

"I think we pediatricians are the only ones in Germany who love the Turks," suggested one pediatrician. There was a touch of romantic hyperbole in his words. But if it was an overstatement, it couldn't have been very far from the truth. In my mailbox that morning I had found a neo-Nazi flyer: AUSLÄNDER STOP. Stop admitting foreigners. Don't let them assimilate, it said. Because they "respected" their culture and religion, this group wanted to see them sent back where they could be fully appreciated.

"Many of our own young people are too pessimistic to become parents," my colleague continued. "Our own birthrate is dropping. We have something to learn from the Turks, what it means to have a heart for children and the courage to continue to bring them into this dangerous world."

Hagar sat between us and her son as we entered the room to make rounds. She was polite and respectful, as was the boy. He was a bright-eyed lad with golden brown eyes that danced. There was hope in those eyes. Ismael knew that he was sick, but he had faith in the German medicine that he would one day study. He believed that we could make him well. His German was limited, but there was promise in his eyes that he would quickly learn.

The tests were all in, and the results clear. Ismael had leukemia, but the sort that holds promise for cure. The treatments in Germany were so successful that American cancer centers were trying them. I was with one of the German oncologists when he went back to the room to talk to Hagar. There were many side effects to the treatment that required explanation.

I watched Hagar as the doctor explained, satisfied that she understood all he said. A foreigner myself, I knew all the alien's tricks. Her German seemed quite adequate. What she lacked in formal education, she more than compensated for with common sense. This was no woman to underestimate.

There was no hospital staff member available who was fluent in Turkish. It fell to Hagar to translate for her son. My colleague worried that she might hold details back, not impart all that he had said. The oncologist pleaded with her to translate it all: The disease was serious, that he might die. The treatment was serious, what he must suffer if he was not to die. And yet, I could see from the look on the child's face that Ismael had heard only good news, not the bad.

The doctor asked again, "Please be sure to tell him everything. Leave nothing out."

She looked at him defiantly. "I've told him all. There is nothing left to say."

I cannot describe Hagar better to you, the emotions that she felt, the pain she confronted. There was a distance, uncommon even in Germany, that she did not wish to bridge. Most of the other mothers on this ward were curious about me, the American anomaly. Not Hagar. Her longings had nothing to do with me. It was as if the kerchief that concealed her hair shut me out from a closer view. Hagar remains for me an intimation, viewed in an antique mirror, dimly.

For the next three days, the chemotherapy was in full force. From morning to night, Ismael was sick. Hagar sat by his side, between us and him. But the days were not all tests and medicine. For a few hours each day, a school teacher came. German textbooks filled Ismael's bedside stand. He was a diligent student, and with his teacher he hunted for the words he sought.

Hagar took time away when the teacher came, the only hour away from his side. His mother was not there that third day of chemotherapy as we made our rounds. His teacher was there, Ismael's fond co-conspirator. She spoke no Turkish, but she understood this bright young man. She stood back as we entered, *Halbgötter in weißen Kitteln*, the white-coated deities.

The youngster had studied us all, wordlessly understood the part that each of us played in this daily drama. Usually, when we made our rounds, Ismael looked first to the most senior doctor, the German professor, the one in charge, but it was my eyes he sought this time. His own eyes were no longer bright and dancing but those of a caged animal. For three days, without warning, he had vomited. It was to a fellow alien that he turned when he begged, "Bitte, nicht mehr." *Please, no more. Have mercy on me and stop all this sickness that I don't understand.*

I was only a visitor there. I never heard the end of Ismael's story, nor Hagar's, but I think about them often. I think of Ismael, choose to believe that he survived, as have so many other children treated in that fine hospital. I think what it must have been like for him to face the chemotherapy without warning. I see his haunted eyes when, back home in America, I meet my newest patient. I slow down in my own explanations these days, take care to clearly communicate.

Ismael would be eighteen years old now, preparing for medical school if he followed his original dream. I imagine his choosing oncology for a career. He seemed so bright and would have so much to offer his patients.

But most of all I think of Hagar, trapped between two cultures, valued by neither. No one at the hospital bore her ill for the way she shielded her son. She did her best even if it was different from our way. No one loved Ismael more than she; no one could have done better. But the foreignness remained.

I thought about them much this year, seven years later. For me, it's another sabbatical year. For Germany, it is the year of Mölln, Rostock, and Solingen: Neo-Nazi gangs, arsonist attacks, and Turkish families burned to death. These extremists may number but a few, but their impact has been devastating. *Can it happen here again?*

Where I lived, hundreds of refugees continued to pour into Germany from every war-torn country in the world. Every week, you noted their increasing numbers on the streets. Would it happen here again? In a bookstore window, I saw a poster framed by a rainbow, a whisper of hope lettered in a modern German hand:

> When an alien resides with you in your land, you shall not oppress the alien. The alien who resides with you shall be to you as a citizen among you. You shall love the alien as yourself. (Leviticus 19:33–34 NRSV)

This ancient mandate from the eternal Law, lost to many in so-called "Christian lands," had been found by a faithful remnant. *The counsel of the LORD stands forever,* I thought, *the thoughts of his heart to all generations. Hagar, the LORD has heard you in your affliction.*

I thought I saw her once in Berlin this year. It was only for a brief moment in a shop on Kurfürstendamm. The woman was smartly dressed, an elegant brown-and-gray scarf accenting a stylish camel coat. She was laughing with a young Turkish man. I could not be certain that it was Hagar and doubted that she would remember me. Was that Ismael with her?

Too late I turned, wanting so to know what had become of them both. But they were gone, and I was left there on Berlin's most fashionable boulevard to imagine what happened to them as aliens in this foreign land.

7

Rahab's Crimson Cord

Then Rahab let Joshua and the spies down by a crimson cord through the window, for her house was on the outer side of the Jericho city wall and she resided within the wall itself. Rahab the prostitute, with her family and all who belonged to her, Joshua spared. Her family has lived in Israel ever since.

JOSHUA 2:15, 6:25 (NRSV)

Rahab lived and worked on the streets from the age of sixteen on. There was a fellowship she found there with other whores. They looked out for each other when no one else would. They were sisters who did not turn their heads away when she walked by.

There were days when she looked like a mannequin on the cover of *Ebony*. When Rahab was feeling well, her skin glowed like a glistening caramel crust, her eyes were fire-bright. But there were those other days—the days that crack seemed to overrule and overwhelm—when people like me might have crossed over to the other side of the street.

Three weeks after she gave birth to the child, Rahab left the baby with a friend. That was how LaVonne became a mother. Rahab was on her way out of town with a guy named Jo Jo. LaVonne suspected that the police were on their trail, the pimp's drug deals about to bust.

Rahab gave her child to a woman who had failed every alcohol rehab program in New Haven County. LaVonne could drink past Antabuse, vomit her guts out, and then keep drinking. One time she kicked a policeman in the butt. He charged her with drunk and disorderly conduct, yet he came to the drunk tank and pleaded with her.

"You're a fine woman, LaVonne," he argued with her. "You don't need this muck. You could make something of yourself. You could be a somebody. Hell, you are a somebody. Why don't you get sober?" Even Sergeant O'Connor (who attended A.A. faithfully himself) finally concluded that LaVonne was hopeless. LaVonne didn't see herself as much different from Rahab. She just had bigger dreams. Sometimes she went to church and sat in a back pew. Those good Christian folks never really looked her square in the eye when she was drunk.

The baby was a tiny thing, nameless as yet. The birth certificate simply read "Female Washington." LaVonne named her "Eva" after the mother of all living. The tiny child she held in her arms could mean a new beginning for them both. It was as if Rahab had thrown a lifeline to her friend. After Eva came into her life, LaVonne went to church regularly. No child of hers would be raised without the songs of her people. For the sake of her new daughter, LaVonne would try.

Long ago LaVonne sang in a gospel choir and would again if they let her. There was an emptiness in her belly that only found filling in God's house. Life had been hard as long as LaVonne remembered. Her people were like the children of Israel, wandering in time and space and ghetto. For LaVonne there had been one Egypt after another, but as long as she never forgot to sing, there would be hope. But she could not abide the preaching about sin.

Sometimes, LaVonne walked out right in the middle of the sermon. She listened to all the fine matrons murmur to each other under the brims of their flowered hats as she passed them by. They covered their mouths with their Bibles, as if she would not know that they were talking about her. But, with Eva, she tried again. She went to church with her baby and held her head high. She was sober in the sanctuary. There was nothing that folks could say about LaVonne when she went to church with her baby.

Motherhood suited LaVonne well. She was up early every morning to bathe and feed her baby, read to her from books. LaVonne became a common sight in the Hill section of New Haven early mornings, strolling with her baby. By 10:00 A.M. they retreated back to the housing project before the drug dealers took over the street and the sound of Uzi fire could be heard. By midday you stayed away from windows and even below them.

LaVonne hadn't heard from Rahab since the day two years earlier that she had casually dropped the baby off. She had heard on the streets that she was in Niantic Women's Prison on a drug charge. Chances were that it was her pimp's sentence that his main lady was serving. Many of the prisoners had been coerced by their pimps or boyfriends to say that the dope was their own. The courts were more lenient with women. She would get out after a shorter sentence and escape a certain beating had she not agreed to take the fall for him. So much for the perks of Rahab's job.

The authorities were never consulted on this "adoption" nor did LaVonne seek welfare money to support the child. She simply took care of the child on her own. There was no way that they would have allowed her to keep the baby, had they known. They would do their own whispering, on paper.

Eva grew up a happy and friendly child whose mother adored, but did not spoil, her. To the staff in Primary Care, LaVonne was known as a reliable mother. No appointment was missed, no baby-shot delinquent. They had no reason to doubt that she was the baby's mother. LaVonne never asked for services that required the birth certificate to be produced. No one in the hospital seemed to notice as long as the baby was healthy.

It was one of the pediatric residents working in Primary Care Clinic who called me. She was worried about Eva because of persistent swollen glands in her neck. A two-week trial of potent antibiotics had not affected them in the least. The child's blood counts were not what they should be for a healthy child. These were all signs that pointed to a malignancy.

LaVonne watched me intently as I examined the child. Nothing fit. The pieces of the puzzle didn't seem to go together for me. I'm sure that I frowned. "You think it leukemia or somepin like that?" she asked. A very good question, since that was exactly what I was checking for.

"I have to tell you that it's a good possibility." I chose my words cautiously. "But none of the tests seems to confirm that. My recommendation is that we check some of that swollen gland under the microscope. It's called a biopsy. That's the next step."

"You gonna cut on ma chil'? I don' want nobody ta cut on ma baby! Ya hear?" And then she began to sob, pressing the child to her.

"It's okay," I tried to reassure her. "You can stay with Eva in the hospital. You can stay with her up to the time she goes into the operating room."

In my innocence, I did not realize the source of her concern. Once the child was in the hospital, once papers needed to be signed, once insurance needed to be checked, LaVonne's secret would be out. Her greatest fear was that the authorities would come and take away her baby.

I cannot say that the child-protection worker was pleased with the arrangement. But they were hard-pressed for foster homes, and the child was temporarily in our care. The biopsy of the lymph node didn't help in the least, and we were left with an enigma. As Eva remained in the hospital, we tried to solve two puzzles. One was her diagnosis. The other was her future. Neither one seemed easy to sort out. As she stayed under our care and test after test came back either negative or hard to interpret, the child's liver and spleen began to swell. Frustrated, I suggested another biopsy, this time the liver. Again, the results were nonspecific. Twice I had to face LaVonne and tell her that we had taken risks but found no answers.

During this time, I noticed that there were two LaVonnes. There was the neatly dressed, bright, caring mother. But there was another LaVonne who missed appointments, especially when the child-protection worker was due. And she rarely stayed at night. The caseworkers seemed to expect only the second LaVonne. But I knew the other, the mother of this child, whose love for her seemed to be worth something.

❧

I suppose it was because the disease was still new that we didn't think of it at first. In fact, AIDS was reported in children for the first time while Eva was going through all the tests for the cancer that she did not have. AIDS was the "gay plague," someone else's problem. No one in the First World seemed to know that it belonged to women and children, too.

Eva was one of the first cases in our hospital. We barely knew what to do with her—or with each other. Was she contagious by simple touch? The infection-control team came once a week, and the rules changed as often.

Signs were hung. They never said that the patient had AIDS, just that there was a risk of "serious" infection. But by that time, most citizens of New Haven knew what type of patient got *Pneumocystis carinii* pneumonia.

Fear came in with the signs. Ultimately, the signs were replaced by supply carts in the hallway by the door. But the dread of the plague did not leave with the plaques.

Something happened to LaVonne when we told her the news. The baby was born to another woman. She had no reason we knew of to fear for herself from the child. She sat looking down at the floor and said the words so quietly that I scarcely heard them. "I done call Nian'ic t'day ta check on 'er. Her mama, she daid."

There were no tears in her eyes, and yet I knew that she cared deeply for this woman. It was no small thing to take in a strange child. There must have been a bond between them.

"LaVonne, are you okay?" I asked. "She was your friend. It must hurt." The tears came.

"It done hurt a lot. She trusted me wit her baby. She be ma friend. She alway' took care a me when I done need takin' care of. Now she daid. Ma baby's mama daid."

She was crying when I came on Sunday afternoon to make rounds. And drunk. "They done kick me out o' church, them sweet life peoples. The elder, he say I go home 'n' sleep or somepin. They don' let me pray for ma baby's mama."

But the elder came that afternoon, prayed with her for Rahab and for her baby. He prayed for LaVonne, that she would follow Jesus and be healed of all her afflictions. LaVonne was there Monday night when I rounded before leaving for the evening. For the first time since the child was admitted, she stayed the whole night. I never saw her drunk again.

LaVonne and Eva had become part of our little landscape. According to the wisdom of the week, the child was to be confined to the room. All those who entered were to gown and glove and mask. As the weeks passed, we realized that we had more advances in rule making than we had in treatment. We didn't have any treatment. But at least for the present time, the child was stable.

We discharged her in LaVonne's care and saw her in the office for follow-up. But I saw LaVonne in the hospital more often than Eva came for outpatient visits. An increasing number of their little family of faith were under our hospital roof. LaVonne prayed with them, reading to them from the Bible.

Afternoons, Elder Edwards went door-to-door on the Hill, a jean-clad simple man, defying the drug lords. He had aged considerably in the last year. It was just a year ago that his only son was taken from him, crossing from the school yard. The hit-and-run joyrider never stopped after he mowed the youngster down. The stolen car was found abandoned later that night.

The boy had been his father's hope, his heir to the ministry. Since early childhood, Terrance never once wavered in his faith. The young man was chosen by God, his father believed. It was the boy who gave the older man the energy to walk door-to-door. When he grew old, his son would be there, in his place. That had been his dream.

His son was gone to Jesus, but the work and the new plague went on. The preacher prayed to the Lord of the harvest to send more laborers into the harvest. And the Lord sent Elder Edwards to the hospital to pray with a poor drunk whose friend had died of AIDS and whose little adopted daughter lay sick with the same illness. He prayed, and LaVonne believed. That was the last day she touched alcohol. LaVonne never looked back.

❧

For a year or so Eva seemed to do all right. Then she was admitted to the hospital for meningitis but quickly recovered. The child was still recovering in the hospital when it happened.

I was on my way to the Emergency Room one night to see a new patient when an ambulance nearly ran me down. They had barely parked when the back doors flew open and two EMTs jumped out with a stretcher. There was a blur of white sheets and black limbs, but staining it all, flowing like a mighty river, was a stream of blood.

On the stretcher was New Haven's latest sacrificial lamb. Hardened to the city's violence, I crossed over to the other side of the driveway and walked toward the pediatric section. Thank God, I did not have to care for adults!

I don't think I would have known until much later if the Edwardses hadn't driven up just then. Sister Edwards went with the stretcher as her husband ran to me. He was shaking so hard that I located two chairs where we could sit in the corridor. I took his hands, felt the jackhammer reverberation of his body in mine.

It was after prayer meeting that night, coming out of the church, that an innocent victim was caught in cross fire.

You didn't even ask why people were shooting anymore. Even the children could tell you it started over drugs.

An anesthesiologist ran by us, joining the Code 12 team. There was an emergency page for a thoracic surgeon. The corridor was a commotion of blurred blue scrub suits, converging on LaVonne's stretcher.

"She was clean, Doc," he sobbed without tears. "She got herself sober. The Lord healed her of all the craving for booze. She was an inspiration to all the folks she visited."

For the longest time, I held his hand and felt his body convulse. The elder was a broken man. His wife came toward us from the direction they had taken LaVonne. There were tears in her eyes. She was shaking her head. A mighty death rattle rose from the throat of the tired holy man. *Let my people go!* he moaned. *Let my people go!*

On the pediatric ward, one of the nurses was cradling Eva in her arms. It was hard to believe that she was once more orphaned. It was our turn to throw a lifeline to a poor motherless child.

Although Eva's legal status as a ward of the court was clarified, no one knew what to do with her. Medically, she was ready to go home, but finding a foster home for her was a different matter. Most of the homes already had other children in them. Were we sure, they asked, that she was not contagious? Could we guarantee the foster mother that she would not get AIDS herself from washing and kissing her? The arguments went on, and Eva remained with us.

It was extraordinary how content she was, staying in her room when asked, without complaint. She did not cry to be embraced but was happy to be held when someone came to her. The child's life attested to the resilience of the human spirit.

We had no idea how long she could live. The nurses—now her mothers—began to decorate her room as if she would be with us for the rest of her life. A shag rug briefly relieved the hospital drab, but the infection-control people pressed for it to be removed. Someone bought Eva a little record player. She loved to play "Ghostbusters" and would invite us to come and dance with her. How she loved to dance! She made my afternoon rounds a joy.

Her chart became thick with so-called progress notes. *The patient is stable. The T4/8 ratio was remeasured and remains unaltered. Blood taken for febrile episode. No source of fever found.* There are many ways to say absolutely nothing.

Between the non-progress notes were intimations of the disaster that would ultimately come to pass. Our bright little daughter was losing her ability to walk and talk. She seemed unable to do things that she easily had done in the previous month. We were learning firsthand about the disastrous consequences of AIDS on the brain of a growing child.

It was during this time that the human immunodeficiency virus was first identified and a test developed. The staff all ran to be tested, most of us using numbers or pseudonyms rather than take the risk that someone might know if we were positive. No one who had cared for Eva had any evidence of the virus. The rules relaxed.

No one found a cure while she was in our care—or since. But progress of another sort did occur. As Eva continued to live on our ward, there was at first a subtle and later more obvious change in the way that decisions were made about her care.

No blood test was drawn, no medication ordered without consulting her nurses. A profound respect replaced the traditional turf wars between doctors and nurses. Any of the senior physicians who came along with a "bright idea" was quickly informed by the house staff that they would do nothing without consulting Eva's primary nurse.

I was on call the last week of her life. For weeks the child's condition had been deteriorating, her liver riddled by an infection that poses no harm to healthy people. She did not leave her bed. As her tummy swelled to accommodate the tumor-like nodules, she refused to eat.

It was on a Sunday afternoon that one of the residents called me back to the hospital. It was obvious that Eva would die the same day. Legally, they needed a note written by the senior attending to let her pass without prolonging her misery.

DNR. *Do not resuscitate*. We had all agreed. The nurses would have it no other way, and they were right. But it was my voice that the state authorities must hear, my pen that must execute our final will and testament for our little daughter. Moments later, she passed from this life in her nurse's arms.

That Sunday seems like a lifetime ago, as if AIDS has been with us forever. Today more than three hundred young children are under care in our hospital for the virus. In our pediatrics department, it is more common than cancer and far more deadly. But there has been progress for children with cancer, and I must believe that the legacy for the children of this new plague will follow.

Years ago, when I started to care for children with cancer, few survived. Neighbor children were sometimes forbidden by their parents to play with my patients with leukemia. It might be contagious by casual contact, mothers told their children. Fear does not demand facts.

Although there is no cure as yet, we are starting to see children with AIDS who are "long-term survivors." We dare to speak of it as a chronic disease. The legacy for the deadly virus's littlest victims will surely follow. That is how we began with cancer. First you survive with a disease, next you outlive it. But the first steps can be the loneliest of all.

Fortunately, these children do not walk alone. A consultant involved in Eva's care left his research laboratory to care for these children, day by day. The community has honored him for his dedication to patients with AIDS. "It's been good for him," his wife told me proudly. "It's been good for his soul."

Eva's primary nurse-mother left the in-patient ward to work full-time with children with AIDS. I hear her silver-bell voice in the clinic and see her eyes sparkle with love and hope as she greets and cares for each of these children.

The state responded to the crisis by developing an effective foster-care program. One woman retired from her nursing career to become a full-time foster mother who takes one child after another into her home and makes them welcome as long as they live. She lays one to rest, and then reaches out to the next.

Eva and LaVonne and Rahab were laid to rest so long ago, yet their legacy lives on through our lives. It is as if, with the child, Rahab passed a lifeline to LaVonne and through her, to us. And the lifeline will continue to be passed as long as there are those who are willing to hold out their hands to receive the precious gift.

Notes

A Window To Heaven

Prologue: Journey to Disbelief

[1]Albert Camus, *The Plague*, translated by Stuart Gilbert (New York: Random House, 1965), 260.

[2]Alan C. Mermann, "Coping Strategies of Selected Physicians," *Perspectives in Biology and Medicine* 33, no. 2 (1990): 2.

Chapter 2: Hearts Unsure, Hearts Untroubled

[1]Dianne Klein, "The Visions of Dying Children Seem to Bring God Alive," *Los Angeles Times, Orange County Edition,* April 22, 1990.

[2]Paul S. Minear, *John, the Martyr's Gospel* (Cleveland, Ohio: Pilgrim Press, 1984), 59.

Chapter 3: Something Better Than Near Death

[1]Klein, "Visions of Dying Children."

[2]Henri J. M. Nouwen, *Letters to Marc about Jesus* (San Francisco: Harper & Row, 1987), 41.

[3]Words and music by C. Austin Miles, Copyright 1912 by Hall-Mack Co.

[4]See Minear, *John, the Martyr's Gospel,* 61.

Chapter 4: A Mystery Story

[1]Sophia Cavalletti, *The Religious Potential of the Child,* translated by Patricia M. and Julie M. Coulter (New York: Paulist Press, 1983).

[2]Henry VanDyke, *The Story of the Other Wise Man* (New York: Harper & Row, 1895).

[3]Jason Gaes, *My Book for Kids with Cansur* (Melius & Peterson, 1989), 42. Jason's parents and the editors of his book had the wisdom to preserve his spelling and grammar and I have followed their example.

[4]Peter Kreeft, *Making Sense out of Suffering* (Ann Arbor: Servant Books, 1986).

Chapter 5: Gifted Clowns

[1]An editorial in the *American Journal of Psychiatry* (99: p. 141) in 1942 argued, "The state of mind of the parents of an idiot may fairly become a subject of psychiatric concern . . . fear of opinion even deters sometimes from placing a mentally deficient child in an institution when the interests of the child and family alike would best be served by such action."

[2]"*Les petite bouffonnes du bon Dieu*" (God's little clowns) is applied to Down's syndrome by Morris West in his wonderful novel, *The Clowns of God* (New York: William Morrow, N. Y. 1981), 336.

Chapter 7: Learning a New Language

[1]Wolf Wolfensberger, "The Prophetic Voice and Presence of Mentally Retarded People in the World Today," an edited presentation to the Religion Subdivision of the American Association of Mental Deficiency at its 100th national conference, Chicago, May 1976.

[2]"The Poignant Thoughts of Down's Children Are Given Voice," *New York Times*, December 22, 1987.

Chapter 8: Angels and Other Strangers

[1]Henri J. M. Nouwen, *Reaching Out; The Three Movements of the Spiritual Life* (New York: Doubleday, 1975), 67, 68.

[2]Richard C. Mouw, *Distorted Truth* (San Francisco: Harper & Row, 1989), 18.

[3]A. J. Solnit, *The Noncustodial Father—An Application of Solomonic Wisdom, in Fathers and Their Families*, ed. Stanley H. Cath, Alan Gurwit, and Linda Gunsberg (Hillsdale, N.J.: Analytic Press, 1989).

Chapter 9: Does Jesus Drive a School Bus?

[1]William F. May, *The Patient's Ordeal* (Bloomington: University of Indiana Press, 1991).

Chapter 10: Surviving the Holocaust
[1]Elie Wiesel, *Messengers of God* (New York: Random House, 1976), 74.

[2]As interviewed on Robert Schuller's television program, "Hour of Power," August 18, 1991.

[3]Viktor Frankl, *Psychotherapy and Existentialism* (New York: Simon and Schuster, 1967), 119.

Chapter 11: Facing Mount Moriah
[1]Frankl, *Psychotherapy and Existentialism*, 25.

[2]Phyllis Trible, "Genesis 22: The Sacrifice of Sarah," Gross Memorial Lecture, Valparaiso University, Valparaiso, Indiana, 1989.

[3]M. Scott Peck, *A Road Less Traveled* (New York: Simon and Schuster, 1978), 17.

Epilogue: Saying Amen
[1]Charles Hummel, *Fire in the Fireplace* (Downers Grove, Ill.: InterVarsity Press, 1978), 89.

[2]Candlelighters is an international organization of parents of children with cancer. The name is taken from the motto, "It is better to light one candle than to curse the darkness."

[3]David B. Biebel, *If God Is So Good, Why Do I Hurt So Bad?* (Colorado Springs: NavPress, 1989), 18.

[4]Ibid.

A Child Shall Lead Them

Prologue: Let Me Tell You About My Grandchildren
[1]This is adapted from a story told by Jack Hayford in an address entitled "Shout for Joy"; Boston, January 1992.

Chapter 2: Let My Heart Be Broken
[1]*American Heritage Dictionary*.

Chapter 3: Isaac's Return from Mount Moriah
[1]Jackie Pullinger with Andrew Quick, *Chasing the Dragon* (London: Hodder and Stoughton, 1980), 224–25.

Chapter 5: Children Who Chisel

[1]Paul S. Minear, *Eyes of Faith* (Philadelphia: Westminster Press, 1956), 14.

[2]Leanne Payne, *The Healing Presence* (Wheaton: Crossways, 1989), 23.

Chapter 6: Converting a Contract into a Covenant

[1]Professor Paul Ramsey quotes here theologian Karl Barth in Ramsey, Paul, *The Patient As a Person: Explorations in Medical Ethics* (New Haven: Yale University Press, 1970).

[2]William F. May, *A Physician's Covenant: Images of the Healer in Medical Ethics* (Philadelphia: Westminster Press, 1983).

[3]Richard E. Peschel and Enid Rhodes Peschel, *When a Doctor Hates a Patient and Other Chapters in a Young Physician's Life* (Berkeley: University of California Press, 1986), 118.

[4]Bernie Siegel, *Love, Medicine and Miracles* (New York: Harper & Row, 1986), 220.

Chapter 8: Hearts Unfolding

[1]"Dartmouth Redesigns Medical Training to Give Future Doctors a Human Touch," *New York Times* (September 2, 1992), B 7.

Chapter 9: The Apple Doll House Parables

[1]Harold H. Wilke, *Creating the Caring Congregation* (Nashville: Abington, 1980), foreword. Dr. Wilke is director of The Healing Community, 138 Alsworth Avenue, New York 10606.

Chapter 10: A Matter of Life and Death

[1]Peter Kreeft, *Love Is Stronger Than Death* (San Francisco: Harper & Row, 1979), xv.

[2]Elisabeth Kübler-Ross, *On Death and Dying* (New York: Macmillan Company, 1969).

[3]Shiela Cassidy, *Sharing the Darkness* (London: Darton, Longman & Todd, 1988), 3. Cf. Luke 4:11–18.

[4]Conrad Hyers, "Easter Hilarity," in *And God Created Laughter: The Bible As Divine Comedy* (Atlanta: John Knox Press, 1987),

24–28. (Quoted by Doris Donnelly in *Divine Folly: Being Religious and the Exercise of Humor, Theology Today*, January 1992, 385–98).

Chapter 12: Beauty by Proximity
[1] 1 Cor. 15:54–55 (NRSV).

Chapter 13: The Color of Pain
[1] Translation of the Mephistopheles libretto by DECCA 1984 Avril Bardoni.

Chapter 14: NIAP Is Pain Spelled Backward
[1] Luci Shaw and Timothy R. Botts, *Horizon-Exploring Creation* (Grand Rapids: Zondervan, 1992), 114.

Chapter 16: Getting Airborne
[1] Browne Barr, *High-Flying Geese: Unexpected Reflections on the Church and Its Ministry* (New York: Seabury Press, 1983), 19.

Epilogue: A Wedding Invitation
[1] Valerie Bell is the author of a book entitled, *Nobody's Children* (Dallas: Word Books, 1989).
[2] May. *A Physician's Covenant*.